D1569892

Mindful
Marijuana Smoking

Mindful Marijuana Smoking

Health Tips for Cannabis Smokers

Mark Mathew Braunstein

ROWMAN & LITTLEFIELD
Lanham • Boulder • New York • London

Published by Rowman & Littlefield
A wholly owned subsidiary of The Rowman & Littlefield Publishing Group, Inc.
4501 Forbes Boulevard, Suite 200, Lanham, Maryland 20706
www.rowman.com

86-90 Paul Street, London EC2A 4NE

British Library Cataloguing in Publication Information Available

Library of Congress Cataloging-in-Publication Data

Library of Congress Cataloging-in-Publication Data
Names: Braunstein, Mark Mathew, 1951-
Title: Mindful marijuana smoking : health tips for cannabis smokers / Mark
  Mathew Braunstein.
Description: Lanham : Rowman & Littlefield Publishers, [2022] | Includes
  bibliographical references and index. | Summary: "Presents in detail ten
  ways to reduce the risks posed by smoking cannabis and examines cannabis
  smoke's potential harm to stained lungs and strained hearts"—Provided
  by publisher.
Identifiers: LCCN 2021051061 (print) | LCCN 2021051062 (ebook) | ISBN
  9781538156674 (cloth) | ISBN 9781538156681 (epub)
Subjects: LCSH: Cannabis—Physiological effect. | Marijuana—Health
  aspects.
Classification: LCC RC568.C2 B73 2022 (print) | LCC RC568.C2 (ebook) |
  DDC 616.86/35--dc23/eng/20211028
LC record available at https://lccn.loc.gov/2021051061
LC ebook record available at https://lccn.loc.gov/2021051062

Contents

Foreword   vii

Acknowledgments   xi

Introduction: Clearing the Smoke from Cannabis   xv

**PART I: HEALTH TIPS: 10 HEALTH HACKS
AND HEALTHFUL SAFEGUARDS**

1   Breathe Easy: Mindful Breathing   3

2   The Ignition System: Playing with Fire   11

3   Joints: Taking an Active Role with Rolling Papers   23

4   Hand Pipes: More than Just a Pipe Dream   37

5   Water Pipes: The Big Bong Theory   47

6   Herbal Vaporizers: Don't Go Up in Smoke   59

7   Seeking Purity: Keeping Your Drugs Off Drugs   79

8   Preserving Potency: Evading Ephemerality   109

9   Water Cure and Green Diet: Every Mouthful Counts   127

10   Don't Worry! When You Light Up, Lighten Up   135

PART II: HEALTH RISKS: THE DOWNSIDE OF GETTING HIGH

11   Cough It Up! Putting Lungs on the Line   141

12   Heartbreaking News: Elevated Blood Pressure
     and Heartbeat   147

Notes   153

Works Cited   177

Index   195

About the Author   207

Foreword

As medical students, doctors have been taught that marijuana is a drug of abuse and a gateway to the use of other harmful, addictive substances. Many years later, I discovered that almost everything I had learned about this plant in medical school was false and that *Cannabis sativa* L. contains a multitude of compounds that have impressive medicinal benefits. Furthermore, I learned that its safety profile far exceeds that of opioids, benzos, and alcohol, as well as many other commonly prescribed pharmaceuticals.

Cannabis has been used as a medicine for thousands of years. Before its prohibition in 1937, for almost ninety years it was listed on the U.S. Pharmacopeia and was used for conditions such as chronic pain, epilepsy, insomnia, menstrual cramps, arthritis, asthma, and a host of other illnesses. Although many accounts suggest that cannabis was used medicinally in ways that didn't involve smoking, for example as tinctures, teas, and edibles, there is evidence that burning and inhaling cannabis was used ceremoniously and perhaps even medicinally by ancient cultures.[1]

Inhalation certainly has advantages in treating severe symptoms that require immediate remedy or in helping some patients reach therapeutic blood levels that are difficult to achieve by other modes of delivery. And it has been speculated that the process of combustion may produce metabolites that are therapeutic and unavailable via vaporization, which may explain why smoking cannabis is the only method by which some patients experience adequate relief.

   While I respect each patient's understanding of what works best for them, as a medical provider I have usually refrained from recommending inhalation, and smoking in particular, as a method of administration for patients with severe symptoms. Instead, vaping flower is an excellent way to achieve nearly immediate relief from cannabis, and it avoids exposure to products of combustion, but it just doesn't work for everyone.

   Interestingly, smoking cannabis has not been found to increase the risk of lung cancer or chronic obstructive pulmonary disease (COPD) as is the case with smoking tobacco. It is speculated that the anti-inflammatory, broncho-dilatory, and anti-tumor effects of the cannabinoids and terpenes in cannabis released in the smoke may counteract the carcinogenic and inflammatory effects of the products of combustion. Or it could be due to the fact that most people do not smoke as much cannabis as they do tobacco. That's not to say that excessive smoking is not damaging to the hair-like cilia in the bronchial tubes, our first line of defense against respiratory infections, or may not lead to other precancerous or cancerous lesions, but to date, it does not appear to increase the risk of lung cancer or COPD.

   When I considered writing a foreword for this book on the art of smoking cannabis, it piqued my curiosity to know more about the mechanics, physics, and science of smoking. In *Mindful Marijuana Smoking*, Mark Braunstein shares a wealth of knowledge on how patients and adult recreational users can maximize the benefits from smoking cannabis while reducing the risk of damaging delicate lung structures through exposure to hydrocarbons, contaminants, tar, and other products of combustion. With many patients utilizing smoking as their delivery method, now I know a lot more about what patients can do to minimize its ill effects.

   The author shares a lot of solid, evidence-based information, and I was not to be fooled by his lighthearted and pun-infused writing style, which made for an easy and enjoyable reading experience. The author's personal journey with medical marijuana and his extensive research

lend to illustrative, real-life examples of what to do and, more importantly, what *not* to do to minimize the potential negative impact that
smoking may have on one's health. He is not just blowing smoke.

Patricia C. Frye, MD
Author of *The Medical Marijuana Guide: Cannabis and Your Health*

Affiliate Associate Professor
Medical Cannabis Science and Therapeutics
University of Maryland
School of Pharmacy

Chairperson, Committee on Education
Society of Cannabis Clinicians

Acknowledgments

Most humble acknowledgments by authors are so exhaustive and lengthy that often they must be relegated to fine print. They might begin with the authors' belated thanks to their beloved first-grade teachers who taught the class the ABCs, and they might end with doting nods to venerable elder colleagues whose tomes had informed or inspired their own research and writing. While my text might not be brief, my list is short. As a teenager during the hippie sixties, for most of my life prohibition had driven my compatriot cannabis connoisseurs to seek the safety of secrecy and anonymity. None are reprobates living on the fringes of society. Rather, some are doctors, lawyers, and professors whose own sense of self-preservation prevailed stronger than mine. Even during our enlightened era of the great plant liberation, many still wish to remain discreet. In contrast, several editorial colleagues were courageous either to have been open about their own fondness for an herbal inebriant or to have been openly receptive to mine.

For admitting me into her cabal of authors a year before the stars aligned to legalize the recreational use of cannabis in both of our states almost simultaneously, I thank my literary agent, Rita Rosenkranz. This book would not have reached the fruition of publication without her.

For sowing a seed, I am indebted to Dale Gieringer, PhD, who edited a stapled and photocopied booklet titled "Health Tips for Marijuana Smokers."[1] Published in 1994, it is a compilation of selected newsletters of the California Chapter of the National Organization for the Reform of Marijuana Laws (NORML). Much of the booklet's unnumbered thirty-five pages actually document the hazards of smoking, something seldom publicized by other cannabis crusaders. Of the eleven pages that actually address ways of minimizing those hazards, Dale's own four-page "Health Tips for Pot Smokers" provides the core. After deliberating over a dozen potential subtitles for my book, I chose the one that paid greatest homage to the cherished seed that Dale had planted.

California voters, including the activist members of its NORML chapter, turned the tide on the losing War on (Some) Drugs when in November of 1996 they legalized medical marijuana. Emboldened by that landmark law enacted on the other end of the continent, I publicly confessed my cannabis crimes in the January 12, 1997, Sunday editorial section of the *Hartford Courant*. Its liberal editors not only accorded my guest commentary the highest honors by placing it on the front page and above the fold, they even commissioned a colorful and unforgettable illustration to fill out the rest of the page. With the publication of "A Connecticut Paraplegic Tells His Story: Marijuana Has Worked the Best in Easing Pain,"[2] I may have risked the wrath of law enforcement, but I no longer had anything left to hide.

While cultivating and nourishing Dale's seedling for the next ten years, I kept notes and saved news clippings for what eventually became my own updated and expanded version of his essay. In 2007, I had the ambitious idea of submitting my nearly completed article to *High Times*, at that time the only cannabis magazine printed south of the Canadian border. The editors never once acknowledged receipt of my article nor of any of my several written follow-ups or phone calls. Alienated by their dead silence but undaunted, I sought a home for my article north of the border in an international medical marijuana magazine, *Treating Yourself: The Alternative Medicine Journal*. Marco Renda, its editor, welcomed my lengthy article, and in 2008 published it with the provocative title, "Getting High and Staying Healthy."[3]

During the next eight years, I kept further notes. While some of the Western states of the United States had newly legalized the recreational use of cannabis, that wildfire had not yet spread to New England. Nevertheless, *Spirit of Change*, a regional New England magazine saw fit to publish a revised and updated version of my article. In 2016, you might expect to find such an article in a stoner or medical marijuana magazine but not in a holistic health journal. Yet Carol Bedrosian was so progressive and supportive an editor that among the articles about yoga asanas, meditation pointers, and raw foods recipes, she published, "First Aid for Cannabis Smokers."[4]

For a second time around, I owe thanks to Dale Gieringer. In a semi-reciprocal half-circle, he generously corrected my book manuscript's errant facts and misconstrued concepts. I hope that upon its publication, Dale will be proud of me as one of his literary heirs.

Mark Mathew Braunstein
Quaker Hill, Connecticut

Introduction

Clearing the Smoke from Cannabis

Cannabis is here to stay. For our own generation, it has never left us. As prohibition is loosening its grip, a rosy dawn is shining a new light upon cannabis. Winding down its fight to suppress a plant that grows like a weed, society is finally learning to live with it. With its social acceptance growing, more of us will be smoking it, and more of us will be admitting it. And for those of us who have long smoked cannabis, it is high time for us to learn how to reduce its health risks because the way that most of us take a hit of pot can also take a hit on our health.

Drugs that we use and might even need provide us with some clear benefits, otherwise we would not use them. But cloaked as side effects, those welcomed rewards also come with unwanted risks. In contrast to the fears of reefer madness portrayed during the twentieth century, nowadays many people view cannabis as harmless. While indeed less harmful than other drugs, cannabis does not come without some hazards. Whether medicinal or recreational, whether herbal or pharmaceutical, whether illegal or legit, all drugs pose risks.

All forms of smoke pose risks. Whether campfire smoke, or burnt toast smoke, or sage smudge stick smoke, all smoke presents health risks. Smoke up a drug, and you've stirred up some double trouble. Cannabis is celebrated as a natural herb, but intentionally inhaling its smoke is inherently an unnatural act that can compromise your physical health. Even as an herbal remedy that can lift your mood and treat a long list of ailments, it is better to not allow its smoke to add another ailment to that list. Smoke in any quantity and from any source irritates s .

the respiratory tract. Smoke is its own smoking gun—without any gun. You might ignore the facts or kid yourself about smoking, but no smoke and mirrors can deceive your lungs. Even incense, which fools the nose, fouls the lungs.

That smoking is bad for your health is old news, but some good news has arrived for most of us. We now can choose from among many alternatives to smoking. Both traditional and innovative methods for delivering the active ingredients in cannabis, called cannabinoids, include processing into alcohol tinctures, oil extracts, flower essences, oral sprays, topical creams, transdermal patches, sublingual strips, time-released capsules, eyedrops, tablets, waxes, salves, and a whole smorgasbord of edibles. Even the cannabinoids themselves, especially tetrahydrocannabinol (THC) and cannabidiol (CBD), have been isolated and concentrated and marketed. As some of us may reside in states or nations whose drug laws are still stuck in the twentieth century, we might be banished from ready access to this treasure trove of more healthful alternatives.

Even when we do have legal access to these alternatives, most of us still prefer to smoke cannabis in its whole and natural form as a dried flower wrapped in a few of its enveloping leaves. Street lingo calls that "bud," short for flower bud. Some of us may prefer the flower simply because we cannot afford the more expensive derivatives and concentrates or the technology required to effectively consume them. Others may prefer smoking because the high or the relief comes on quickly, within just a minute or two. When you so promptly know you've had enough, you can easily avoid having too much. And too much of a good thing is rarely a good thing.

So we continue to puff on joints or pipes or herbal vaporizers. The traditional bud form thus outsells all other cannabis products available in dispensaries and pot shops alike. And in the underground marketplace, flower power reigns supreme. One survey published in 2016 found that nine out of ten adults who imbibed still preferred the herbal form of cannabis.[1] Another published in 2020 yielded similar results.[2] If it were a television ad, its off-camera narrator would announce, "Four out of every five cannabis consumers recommend smoking or vaping dried herb over all other methods of delivering cannabinoids."

In the same tradition of dilution and moderation, those who consume alcohol drink more beer and wine than they do hard liquors. If you get high by smoking cannabis, you already are thinking outside the bottle. While it's safe to say that cannabis is safer than alcohol, that's like comparing apples with Agent Orange. A more fitting analogy is comparing smoking cannabis with smoking oregano. Eating oregano is safe, but smoking it is not. Like tough love or square circles, healthful smoking is an oxymoron. If smoke you must, you can take precautions to render smoking less harmful.

For lifelong smokers, after many years the act itself can become a ritual that is difficult to relinquish despite all the alternative forms now available to us. As hardcore holdouts, we might merrily cling to our Luddite ways. Whether you are a patient or a pothead, a tenderfoot toker or a seasoned smoker, a dabbling dilettante or a cannabis connoisseur, if your preferred method of partaking is smoking, then this book is for you.

So, in part I, we will consider in detail no less than ten ways to reduce the health risks posed by smoking cannabis. Then in part II, as an afterthought to reducing those risks, we'll briefly examine cannabis smoke's potential harm to strained hearts and to stained lungs.

Are you ready to safeguard your health by learning a new way of smoking?

Part I

HEALTH TIPS: 10 HEALTH HACKS AND HEALTHFUL SAFEGUARDS

Chapter One

Breathe Easy

Mindful Breathing

To reduce any health risk of smoking cannabis, the number one safe-guard is also the easiest. You do not need to reach into your first-aid kit for this, nor need you do anything more than what you already are doing. Actually, you need to do less. So, if you read no further than the next paragraph, read only that.

Once you inhale the smoke or the vape, do not hold it in! It's that simple. When you hold your breath, you put your health on hold. This will be on the quiz, so pay attention. Don't hold your breath!

DON'T WASTE YOUR BREATH

Holding in your breath longer than you otherwise do when not smoking does not make you any higher. The doctors in the white coats have even analyzed this. Scientific studies have proven that holding your breath is a waste of your time and quite a waste of your breath. So don't waste your breath. Don't hold that hit!

It's no coincidence that, if you cough, it's usually on that hold. So breathe naturally and normally, almost as though you were not smoking. Inhale and exhale casually, without fanfare or deliberation. Even tobacco smokers, who may sometimes inhale long and deep drags, rarely hold it in.[1] If they always held their breath the way that most cannabis smokers do, tobacco smokers would all be dead. So take it easy and breathe easy!

3

When your shaman or mentor or older sibling turned you on as an initiate to the rite of smoking cannabis, your cannabis coach probably instructed you to inhale deeply and to hold that toke. Such an unfamiliar and unnatural way of breathing may have contributed to your failure to get high on that first try or two. In 1992, while campaigning for the presidency, Bill Clinton admitted that during his college years, "I experimented with marijuana a time or two, and I didn't like it. I didn't inhale."[2] This seems unlikely. Instead, he should have claimed that he *couldn't* inhale. Clinton might have failed because the forced technique of intentionally inhaling smoke and then holding it in was so unnatural to him. It's unnatural and contrary to normal human physiology for all of us, too.

COUGH IT UP!

Here comes an anatomy lesson with some physiology thrown in. So, if the mere thought of peeking into your innards makes you feel queasy, consider skipping this section. Or just close your eyes, and I'll let you know when it's over. This won't be on the quiz.

Once you fill your lungs with smoke-filled air, holding your breath will not result in any further absorption of the cannabinoids,[3] nor in any further enhanced psychoactive or medicinal effect. Cannabinoids are fat-soluble and so are quickly absorbed within the lungs. "Tars" is a diffuse term for the hydrocarbons produced by the combustion of plant matter. Tars are not fat-soluble, so are absorbed more slowly. More than any contaminants or debris in smoke, tars muck up the works. Holding your breath only promotes more intake of tars and therefore more irritation to your lungs.

The literary scion Aldous Huxley rhapsodized about the psychedelic drug experience in his 1954 classic *The Doors of Perception*. The rock band, the Doors, embraced their name in an homage to that book's title. For the cannabis drug experience, cannabinoids enter through the doors of the lungs. Think of your lungs as two huge playing fields with several main players, all on the same team—your team. For our discussion, the star athletes are the alveoli cells, the goblet cells, and the cilia cells.

Alveoli cells are tiny air sacs lining the interior membranes of the lungs. They absorb oxygen to assimilate it into the bloodstream. Absorption of oxygen is by design, while absorption of other miscellaneous substances is by accident. Cannabinoids just happen to be among the miscellanea that catch a ride with the oxygen.

While the alveoli are the doorways, goblet cells and cilia cells are the doormats. You wipe your feet on a doormat, so you won't track dirt into your home.

Goblet cells secrete mucus to trap tars, ash, and other gunk to prevent them from being tracked into your bloodstream. Cilia cells are delicate hair-like hooks that scrap away that schmutz-clogged mucus to move the schmutz back up the hatch. Cilia cells can become overburdened by an overload of smoke or foul air, regardless of the origin. If too gummed up to do any further heavy lifting, the cilia slacken at their job. Mucus then accumulates in your lungs. Pathogens lurking about and hanging out in the primordial soup in your lungs then flourish and multiply. And whammo!—you come down with a cold, the flu, an acute case of bronchitis, or a not so cute case of pneumonia. Thus, heavy cannabis smokers compared to nonsmokers have garnered a well-deserved reputation for succumbing to more episodes of respiratory illnesses.[4] Try your best to cough it up and get it out.

If you can't cough up phlegm but fruitlessly just keep on trying, yours becomes a hacking cough. If you suppress that hacking cough with syrups or lozenges, you are treating only the symptom but not the cause of the cough. Granted, breathing urban air or occupying a toxic building can also be the root of your wheezing, coughing, or spitting. While not everyone is fortunate enough to be able to choose where to live or to work, we all can take control of whether or how to smoke cannabis.

So if you often find yourself wheezing, coughing, or spitting, that's probably because you hold it in too long. Nurture your inner child by sparing your inner lungs. When you smoke or even when you vape, don't hold your breath.

Health Tip for All Smokers and Vapers of Either Tobacco or Cannabis: Once you inhale the smoke or vape, don't hold your breath.

A BREATHTAKING EXPERIENCE

Several medical studies have proven that trying to enhance the effects of cannabis smoke by holding your breath is ultimately a waste of your time and a waste of your breath. The first was conducted in 1989,[5] another in 1991,[6] a third in 1992,[7] and a fourth in 1995.[8] Since then, both cannabis advocates and medical doctors have advised potheads and patients alike, yet their words have seemingly fallen on deaf ears.

Mitch Earleywine, PhD, a psychology professor and an author and editor of several scholarly books about cannabis, has publicized the futility of the deeply held but mistaken belief about holding in your smoke.[9] When he has warned about this in public lectures, some unreceptive members of his audiences have displayed not just healthy skepticism but downright hostility. They have hurled things at him, and the projectiles were not mere spitballs or rotten tomatoes.[10] As a lectern does not provide much cover, his must have been a breathtaking experience.

THE SMOKE-KISS

But wait! There have been special occasions when I did indeed hold that hit. The only logical reason for holding your breath is to use those extra moments to get into position for sharing your breath. Call it the "smoke-kiss." Expressed in the vernacular, the smoke-kiss is known as "shotgunning" or as a "shotgun kiss," but those misbegotten monikers have long been overdue for overhauls.

If you are impoverished, frugal-minded, or just plain cheap, you can save on the high cost of cannabis by recycling your second-hand smoke. Share it with your significant other(s). Exhale while kissing them, while they likewise inhale while kissing you. As a bonus, your recipients will benefit by having the burning hot smoke cooled down to body temperature. If they happen to be inexperienced newbies, harsh smoke will not be as hard on their tenderfoot lungs, and they will be less prone to coughing it out.

Acting with altruism in your heart and purely the interests of science in your mind, conduct a practice session. You likely will find that not only does sharing your second-hand smoke get both of you equally high or equally medicated, it will even add a touch of romance and intimacy into your relationship.

HYPOXIA AND HYPERVENTILATION
AND HUFFING AND PUFFING

Some diehard smokers swear by the practice of holding their breaths because they consider lightheadedness to be part of their high. Holding your breath, with or without smoke, causes a reduction of oxygen reaching your brain. The havoc wreaked upon your brain cells is called hypoxia. Even without smoking, if you hold your breath long enough, the oxygen deprivation will make you feel giddy or dizzy. You might experience the same sensation from choking on a chunk of meat, from coughing up a lungful of phlegm, or from drowning in a pool of water.

It is our human nature to seek altered states of consciousness. Even as children, many of us made ourselves giddy by performing multiple somersaults down a hillside. Or we made our heads spin by standing and whirling our bodies around in circles. As a form of play, we enjoyed the dizziness and loopiness that the whirling produced. As adults, some Sufi dervishes do this as a form of prayer, chanting, and meditation, all rolled into one.

Hyperventilation, too, will make you feel lightheaded. As an adult, you might try huffing and puffing like the Big Bad Wolf blowing down the house of one of the "Three Little Pigs." "I'll huff and I'll puff and I'll blow your house down!" Go ahead and knock yourself out, though while you're at it you might kill off a few thousand brain cells. At least by not huffing and puffing with smoke in your lungs, you won't be damaging any lung cells.

THE BREATH OF LIFE

Some smokers firmly believe that, until they cough, they will not have inhaled enough smoke to make them high. They anticipate the coughing as their signal that they have smoked enough. Actually, coughing signals that they have smoked too much. While coughing expands the lungs, that is only because it has irritated them. Taking long and deep tokes and holding it in, too, expands the lungs. But because smoke is in the mix, the size of the lungs is a measure only of quantity, not quality.

For a more healthful way of expanding lung capacity, try improved techniques of breathing. Yogis, free divers, singers, and wind instrumentalists practice it. You can read entire books that are just devoted to teaching you how to breathe deeply. Or you can get off your butt and find joy in your body. Try engaging in some physical exercise, especially aerobics such as walking, swimming, rowing, biking, running, and dancing. Try just about any activity except staring into cellphones or reading books or sitting around smoking a joint.

DIY ANIMAL EXPERIMENTATION

Unconvinced by the above advice not to hold your breath? Okay, go ahead and conduct some animal experiments, the animal being you.

Phase 1

1. First, clear your head. If you're a recreational user, don't toke for at least forty-eight hours.
2. Measure two equal quantities of your favorite stash into two doses, dosage A and dosage B.
3. Sit back, relax, and switch on one of your favorite pieces of music. Take your time. This is not a race.
4. Administer dosage A in the way you usually smoke—if that means taking long drags, then holding your breath and then slowly exhaling. Keep count of your tokes. If you lose count, you'll just have to start all over again. (Only kidding!) Else ye olde short-term memory loss kicks in and you forget that number, write it down.
5. Also make note of how you feel. If you're a medicinal user, have you relieved your symptoms? If you're a recreational user, are you as high as a kite?

Phase 2

1. First, clear your head. If you're a recreational user, don't toke for the same time period that you had waited before conducting Phase 1.
2. At the same time of day as before, sit back, relax, and listen to that same music or, if you cherish your antique collection of vinyl LPs, listen to side B.

3. Administer dosage B, but this time not in your usual way. Instead, toke up without taking long drags and without holding your breath. Inhale and exhale the same as you would when not thinking about it, even though this time you will be thinking about it.
4. Repeat until you are all out of dosage B, again keeping count of your tokes and writing it down. If it matches the number from your previous session, all the better.
5. Also take notes about how you feel.

Compare your notes. Is the relief or the high the same? If so, Your Honor, I rest my case. If not, then a lifetime of smoking in your traditional manner might have been a hard pattern to change after years or even decades of conditioning. You might have messed up on step 3 of Phase 2. If you still are skeptical, proceed with some more "animal" testing.

THE HYPOXIA HYPOTHESIS

Further experimentation is reserved for smokers who are dead set on holding their breath. Research has shown that cannabis smokers will experience the same boost to their high by simply holding in a placebo of air.[11] Conduct Experiment Number 2, modeled upon a novel idea suggested by Professor Earleywine.[12] As a variation of Phase 2, first exhale the cannabis smoke and then hold your breath. Compare notes. I'd be very interested in learning your results. I might find it reassuring to know that others in this world besides myself are blowing a lot of hot air.

Chapter Two

The Ignition System
Playing with Fire

After learning in chapter 1 that there is a better way to inhale, time now to seek a new way to ignite. Otherwise, when you fire up your herb, you might inhale the noxious fumes of the butane lighter or the match head.

WHAT YOU SMELL IS WHAT YOU BREATHE

Countless medical studies have shed light upon the health risks of smoking herbs, be they tobacco or cannabis. However, apparently no research has examined the risky business of inhaling the ignition fumes from lighters or matches. As no one has thought to conduct studies to prove it, researchers must hold as self-evident that such fumes should be avoided. Meanwhile, the absence of any studies offers no excuse for our hiding behind a smokescreen of denial. Rather, deductive reasoning should convince us that the foul odors emitted by lit lighters and struck matches must be unsafe to breathe. And if you're smelling them, then you're breathing them.

Typically, tobacco smokers light up just once per pre-rolled commercial cigarette. Chemical additives to control the burn rate of the tobacco account for that one-match wonder.[1] When we roll our own homemade joints, sometimes imperfectly, and we smoke cannabis without such additives, we often need to light up each joint more than once. When we smoke pipes, be it a hand pipe or a water pipe or a bong, we may need to fire it up several times. As the cumulative ignition fumes for every joint or pipeful of cannabis pose more risks than per tobacco cigarette, it is high time that we explore bright new ideas for tuning up our ignition systems.

TRIAL BY FIRE

As a natural fiber with no chemical additives, a twig will pose fewer risks than a lighter or a match. If you happen to stand near a roaring campfire or fireplace, you can remove a twig that is burning on only one end and apply its flaming tip to your joint or pipe. Impractical but possible. Of course, you first must find some kindling and then must employ one of four odorless ways to spark it ablaze:

1. Find two sticks. Rub the sticks together so that their friction generates heat.
2. Get out a magnifying glass. Train the rays of the noonday sun through the lens to pinpoint those rays.
3. Buy a spark wheel. You get several rods of ferrocerium flint. One inserts into a brass mount on which spins a steel flywheel, same as in many cigarette lighters, minus the butane.
4. Buy a magnesium fire starter. You get a set of two or three tiny tools compact enough to carry on your keychain: a magnesium rod, a ferrocerium flint, and a steel striker. Often the flint is embedded along the magnesium rod, so totaling only two tiny tools.

Mastering any of these odorless techniques for starting a fire can be daunting and reserved only for the brave. You can enlist the services of a Boy Scout, if any are around. Or enroll in a survivalist retreat. Or participate in an historic reenactment of *The Flintstones* cartoon. Or for the sake of convenience, you can join the rest of society and resort to the labor-saving devices of matches and lighters.

THE UNMATCHED HAZARDS OF MATCHES

The more common matches are called "safety matches," the word "safety" distinguishing them from less common "strike-anywhere matches."

Strike anywhere matches contain potassium, phosphorus, sulfur, and perchlorates, all combined into one match head. If you are not up to snuff on your incendiaries and pyrotechnics, you may not know that perchlorates are also used in missile fuels, explosives, flares, and fireworks. Stand anywhere within their striking distance and you will be painfully aware of the foul smell of the plume of strike anywhere matches. Even minding their own business while quietly sitting in the box, they smell toxic.

Although legal, strike anywhere matches are highly flammable, so most shipping carriers either ban their transport or tack on hefty hazmat surcharges. Due to high shipping costs, many manufacturers have discontinued making them, so you will seldom find strike anywhere matches sold in everyday grocery stores. If you insist, look for them in outdoor sporting goods stores where they are marketed for starting campfires. By tacking on the hazmat shipping surcharge to the base cost of the product, online merchants do sell them, but at ten times the price of standard safety matches.

Safety matches are "strike-on-box matches." The sulfur and highly flammable phosphorus are removed from the match head. Instead, they are placed into the striking surface of the ugly-brown strips that adhere to the sides of matchboxes or matchbooks. Safety matches indeed are safer because the phosphorous and sulfur ignite only minimally and do not fill the air with their toxic fumes.

Matchboxes and *matchbooks* both present other perils. Hold the matchstick for too long and—ouch!—you burn your fingers. Numerous studies have proven that burns are not conducive to good health. Also, wooden matchsticks of matchboxes are prone to break when struck, while paperboard matchsticks of matchbooks easily drop from your grasp while lit. As fire hazards, both types of matches are unmatched.

Health Tip for How to Use Matches: Once you get that match going and are ready to fire up your herb, be wary of that first toke! In theory, you can wait for the flaming match head to burn out and then apply only the burning shaft to your herb. In practice, that toxic glowing ember smolders as the shaft burns down perilously close to your fingertips. Conveniently, hot air rises. While you wait for that match head to fully extinguish, you can avoid inhaling match head fumes by holding the match above your head.

MAKING SPARKS WITH SPARK LIGHTERS

Flicking a lighter fills the air with less noxious fumes than does striking a match, so it's a relief that we can avail ourselves of the modern
convenience of lighters. Spark lighters fueled by butane are pocket-size,
which accounts for their widespread use. Cheaper disposable lighters
designed to fit inside a pack of cigarettes are sparked by ferrocerium
flint, while more expensive non-disposable models are sparked by piezo
quartz.

Flint lighters require you to flick the serrated steel flywheel with your
thumb. After many flicks, the tip of your thumb will form callouses or
abrasions. When you flick the flywheel, here called a spark wheel, you
spin the spark wheel that scrapes the ferrocerium flint inserted below
the wheel, which creates a spark. True flint stone had been used to spark
cigarette lighters until the twentieth century. Present day flint is actually
ferrocerium, a hazardous metal. When sparked, faux-flint lighters create
a toxic cloud of microscopic ferrocerium dust resembling a tiny puff of
smoke. Bad timing if you inhale at the same time that you flick.

Health Tips for How to Use Flint Lighters: To allow the ferrocerium
dust to settle, wait two seconds before holding the flame to your joint.
Forget about these for pipes. The flame from a flint lighter, like from a
candle, only rises upward. Try to toke from the bowl of a short-stemmed
pipe and you suck in the flame. Beware that yellow flame! Probably
worse, because you are holding the lighter sideways, that yellow flame
sometimes extinguishes while you are still inhaling, presenting the risk
of inhaling incompletely combusted butane fumes. Hold the lighter only
in an upright position.

Piezo lighters are sparked by quartz crystals that create an electrical
charge by mechanical stress. They eliminate the toxicity of faux flint.
Also known as torch lighters, jet lighters, barbeque lighters, or cigar
lighters, they have adjustable and windproof flames that can be aimed
sideways and even upside-down. Like miniature blowtorches with long
and pivotable throws, piezo lighters are ideal for firing up pipefuls of
cannabis. In fact, when designed for pipes, they are called pipe lighters.

Some flint lighters provide a tremendous improvement in the mecha-
nism of a lever that flicks the spark wheel for you. The lever resembles
the quieter push button on piezo lighters, but it is not the real thing, as
its true identity is divulged by its loud click. The flame is still lame, as

it rises only upward. Such flint lighters are only masquerading as wannabe piezo lighters.

Health Tip for How to Use Piezo Lighters: Ignited by a push button rather than a spark wheel, piezo lighters are kind on both your thumb and your lungs. While more expensive than flint lighters, piezo lighters are relatively safer especially when used on pipes, making them worth their extra cost. Same as flint lighters, piezo lighters are fueled by butane. Beware butane.

BUTANE-FUELED LIGHTERS

With the notable exception of Zippo brand lighters that are fueled by liquid naphtha or a naphtha spin-off, butane is the most common fuel for cigarette lighters. Stored under pressure inside the lighter, butane is liquid. Once released from the lighter, the liquid turns into a colorless gas with a very faint but unpleasant odor, though some people consider it odorless. Intentionally inhaling that gas can prove fatal.[2]

As a hydrocarbon, butane fumes are both toxic and intoxicating. Some foolish little kiddies, desperate to get high, intentionally sniff the fumes from butane cannisters. Small-dose short-term effects include headache, dizziness, and coughing. Long-term effects from repeated use include kidney, liver, heart, and brain damage.[3] Note that the direst effects are from fumes straight from the liquid butane cannister. Many scientific studies have measured the toxicity of butane fumes as a recreational inhalant, but none measure the toxicity of lighters when lit. No study even attempts to account for the absence of such studies. An important principle taught to law students in law school is that the absence of evidence is not evidence of absence. This omission by researchers is akin to studying the fumes emitted from the nozzle of a gasoline pump but not from the exhaust from the tailpipe of a truck.

More sober-minded adults do not use butane directly from the liquid-filled cannister. We use butane only from a lighter in order to fire up our herb. Over time, infrequent and brief use might expose us to cumulative toxic effects. If we suck in the fumes from the combustion of butane, our first toke may be more harmful than the whole rest of the joint or pipeful of combusted cannabis. Until we can read a scientific study about the cumulative effects of long-term use of lighters, we instead can read the labels affixed to butane lighters. The fine print on the lighters issue several warnings: "Warning! Contains flammable gas under pressure."

Unlike metal lighters, cheap plastic lighters have been known to explode if exposed to external heat. Also stated on their labels, "Warning! Never expose to heat above 50°C (122°F) or to prolonged sunlight." The cheapest lighters are so faulty that their flames do not always fully extinguish after you've removed your finger from its lever, so "Warning! Be sure flame is completely out after every use." That lever can be so tiny and quirky that it requires effort to keep it depressed, easily irritating your thumb tip, so "Warning! Do not keep lit for longer than 30 seconds."

Refillable metal lighters are more expensive and more dependable, but refilling them can be messy and risky, and the vents for refueling pose a danger of leakage. Which lighter is safer? Plastic and disposable? Or metal and refillable? How about which of Ulysses' passageways is safer? Scylla or Charybdis?

Health Tip for How to Use Butane Lighters: Never press on the lever without sparking it, because then you are releasing butane fumes into the very air you are breathing. If you are a skeptic bent on self-destruction, try pressing the lever while placed right under your nostrils. Then take a whiff. That's what some silly little children would do, so keep lighters out of reach of children. As for adults, go light on your use of lighters.

FLAMELESS LIGHTERS

Flameless lighters were first called Tesla lighters, as they were based upon the Tesla coil, one of Nikola Tesla's many inventions. In 1891, the first Tesla coil was bigger than an elephant. The pocket-size Tesla lighter is now smaller than a mouse.

The Tesla lighter has been dubbed with a variety of descriptive names such as electronic lighters, electric-arc lighters, electronic-coil lighters, plasma-beam lighters, and many combinations in between. Nowadays almost all get juiced on USB charges, so add USB lighter to its list of aliases. All are buzzwords for the same dang thing. While "plasma" sounds like something living and "electric-arc" adds the allure of hi-tech hocus-pocus, here we'll settle on "flameless" to better distinguish it from the more common flame-emitting butane lighter.

Flameless lighters are windproof and, when capped, some are waterproof. With no liquid or gas fuel that might escape, they are leakproof. Their on/off switches, unlike those on butane lighters, are all easy on your thumb. Free of chemicals and odors, they eliminate the toxicity of both flint and butane. While they generally cost more than refillable butane lighters, they cancel out the extra expense of that sinister cannister of butane fuel, so they potentially can cost less.

No fuel, no flame, no fumes, no smoke—unfortunately, absent from this list is "no problem." The technology is still in its infancy. Thomas Edison did not invent the lightbulb, but he did perfect it. The flameless lighter has yet to be perfected. There are no eternal flames, and no flameless lighters last forever. Even mid-priced models remain functional for barely one year. Over time, charges do not last as long, and recharging takes longer. Their nonreplaceable lithium-ion batteries, like all rechargeable batteries, will die. Anticipating that few people would bother taking the time and paying the postage to return defunct lighters with dead batteries, some manufacturers do offer warranties, some spanning several years. When the batteries die, you are left with a nonrecyclable piece of junk. Rather than to be left dry and not high, seek models that feature LED lights that indicate the level of the battery charge. User hint: buy two lighters. One will serve as a backup while you recharge the other one, or when that other one dies.

Press the on/off button or slide its switch, and the coil emits an arc-shaped spark that dances between two electrodes. The coil also emits a faint, high-pitched crackling hiss that is imperceptible to some human ears. Other people with sharp hearing can detect the hiss from several paces away. While not a health hazard, the sound can be irritating to those who can perceive that high frequency. Cats more than dogs are known to become agitated by its sound. Turned on near a radio, it can cause static interference with the radio's signal. If your radio transmits the music of the spheres, your flameless lighter emits the static of the spheres.

Think of its spark as a pocket-size bolt of lightning. Place your joint into the arc of the spark, and your joint ignites. Because the housing or the flip cap can get in the way, the arc of many flameless lighters cannot reach the contents inside the bowl of a pipe. That's a job for flameless torch lighters.

Rather than single-coiled, flameless torch lighters are double- or triple-coiled. The bowls of pot pipes are smaller and shallower than those of tobacco pipes, so smaller torch lighters that make no claim about being suitable for tobacco pipes often will work fine for pot pipes, and that includes bongs and water pipes. Larger torch lighters that go by the name "pipe lighter" are good for tobacco and cannabis alike.

Never apply a torch lighter to a metal pot pipe, as it might shock you with a mild electrical impulse. Still, you might get some jollies from such shocking experiences, like those you might remember from grade-school science experiments while generating static electricity.

Health Tip for How to Use Flameless Lighters: Compared to butane, the ignition of rechargeable flameless lighters is eco-friendly. Emitting no detectable odor, they are safe to inhale. No flames, so no fumes. Ditch the flick of your Bic. The flameless lighter just might light the way to the future.

CHOOSE YOUR WEAPON

Match or lighter? Striking a match fills the air with more noxious fumes than does flicking any lighter, so you would think that lighters always win over matches. Not so fast! A match can be an appropriate tool when you're lighting up a pipe rather than a joint. So the first question to ask is, joint or pipe?

Health Tip for How to Light Up Joints: With your two hands occupied striking a match, you must hold a joint in your mouth, where you can't avoid inhaling ignition fumes. In contrast, with your one hand flicking a lighter and the other holding the joint, you can hold both at arm's length, so far enough away to minimize your exposure to the ignition fumes of a lighter. To more safely light up a joint, look to lighters.

Health Tip for How to Light Up Pipes: Unless the pipe stem is more than a foot (30 cm) long, when lighting the bowl, you're holding that flame right in front of your nose. Smoked leisurely, especially during solo sessions, cannabis snuffs out easily, requiring several firings per bowl. That's toxic buildup. Nix to matches and cheap lighters that force you to suck in that flame. When smoking a pipe, the safer ignition system is the piezo lighter that can aim its flame sideways or downward, and the safest of all is the flameless pipe lighter.

THE FIRE POWER OF CANDLES

But wait! You can still safely use a match or a cheap flint lighter. Strike just one match or hit one flick, not to light your pipe, but to light a candle. Candles, preferably made with a wax other than paraffin, can be true drug paraffin-alia!

Candles are made from a variety of ingredients, including paraffin, tallow from animal fats, vegetable oils often from palm, soy, or coconut, and beeswax. Hold a white sheet of paper or board high above a burning candle, and it won't stay white for long. You will capture a coating of soot, which is mostly carbon ash. Soot is only what you happen to see. Hidden to the naked eye, the candle's fumes also contain, for instance, carbon monoxide,[4] volatile organic compounds (VOCs),[5] and PAH.[6] Polycyclic aromatic hydrocarbons, called PAH for short, are produced during incomplete combustion. (For more about PAH, see chapter 7.)

As a petroleum distillate, paraffin is plentiful, cheap, and potentially the most harmful, as its fumes contain phthalates. Phthalates consist of an enormous class of chemical plasticizers. Whenever one is studied in a common household product, it is always found to be harmful to human health.[7] Health food, new age, and occult stores sell vegetable oil candles that are labeled as free of phthalates. Soy candle manufacturers claim that their candles not only emit no phthalates, but also the least amount of soot. In order to avoid exposure to the tortured spirits of factory farm animals, practitioners of Wicca avoid candles made of tallow, which is an animal fat. Adherents to kosher dietary laws also shun tallow when their candles are intended for religious observance. Such candles are labeled K for kosher.

Despite the ubiquitous use of candles since the dawn of human history and even into our present age, only a few studies have evaluated the emissions from burning candles.[8] One study has shown that added scents of any kind add to the candles' pollutants.[9] Another study has compared the pollutants from the fumes of commonplace paraffin compared only to beeswax. Beeswax proved to be far less polluting.[10] In effect, paraffin cannot hold a candle to beeswax.

Most recently, a study published in 2021 evaluated both waxes and fragrances, specifically four sources of waxes and five types of fragrances.[11] The four sources of wax were palm oil, soy oil, tallow, and paraffin, while omitting beeswax. In all cases, the candles without any scents produced far lower toxic emissions than those with scents.[12] Fragrance-free palm oil had the lowest emissions, fragrance-free soy oil rated a very close second, fragrance-free tallow had more, and fragrance-free paraffin the most of the four.[13] While we know from an earlier study that fragrance-free beeswax is safer than fragrance-free paraffin, we do not know where on the scale of pollutants does beeswax compare to palm oil or soy oil. Candle researchers, are you listening?

Wicks, too, pose health risks. While made of flammable fibers, wicks have metal cores to slow their burning and to enhance their vertical shape. Most candles made in North America contain wicks with zinc cores, which is considered safe. Most candles made in China contain wicks with lead cores, which should be shunned.[14] If made with lead, the burning wicks release toxic lead into the air.[15] Beware the Wicked Wicks of the East.

When burning candles are smothered or blown out, their wicks smolder and emit lots of soot and foul odors. Snipping the wick with scissors is the most effective way to produce the least amount of smolder when snuffing out a candle.[16]

By now you must rightfully be wondering, why even bother lighting it? Compared to repeatedly flicking butane lighters or striking matches, lighting a candle only once does have something to commend. You can place your burning candle at arm's length, so you are out of range from its fumes. In the candle's flame, you can stoke up a glass wand, a hemp wick, or a toothpick. Then to toke your pipeful, apply that glowing wand, that smoldering wick, or that burning toothpick. No toxic plume in your face, so none in your lungs.

Glass wands are also called weed wands. Glass wands may make sense in theory, but in practice they involve risk of singeing your fingers and pose a potential fire hazard. The theory is that you heat the tip of a thin borosilicate glass rod, and then insert it into the herb, more like scorching rather than simply igniting the herb. Decorative glass rods intended for mixing alcoholic drinks are too thick to heat up readily. Instead, fragilely thin glass wands sold specifically for igniting cannabis fit the bill.

Danger, however, lurks after using that scorching wand just when you want to remain relaxed after toking. Good luck on placing the cylindrical wand somewhere safe so it won't roll away, ignite a conflagration, and cause a house fire. Some stoner websites sing praises for glass wands but overlook the high risk of singeing your fingers or burning your house down.

Hemp wicks are spools of hemp twine coated with beeswax. Once ignited, they burn down slowly just like the wick of a beeswax candle. Are they metallicized same as the wicks of candles? Manufacturers make no claims to the contrary. Igniting cannabis with hemp fiber makes sense. It is a romantic notion that has inspired many a smoker to give it a try. But in between tokes, when it is not in use, you must keep a watchful eye on the flimsy and cumbersome burning hemp wick or else it can ignite the entire spool. This is yet another unnecessary fire hazard.

The hemp wick is an invention that may have originated in the wildest daydreams of a stoner who was stoned. It somehow gets promoted without any advisories by cannabis news websites as a viable alternative to matches and butane lighters. You definitely should be wary—for hemp enthusiasts only.

Toothpicks are safer substitutes for glass wands and hemp wicks. Thin flat toothpicks burn truer than thicker round ones. Go for flat, not round, toothpicks. Flat toothpicks easily ignite in the flame of that candle, and then readily stay lit long enough for you to fire up your pipe. Toothpicks also prove very handy for stirring the contents of your bowl. Costing less than hemp wicks, an inexpensive box of toothpicks will last you many dozens of smoking sessions.

Health Tip for How to Light Up Pipes: Using an unscented candle made of beeswax or vegetable oil, light it and then place it at arm's length, so you are out of range of its fumes. Hold a flat toothpick by its broad end and place its narrow end into the flame. Now light up the bowl of bud—wood, a natural fiber, to the rescue.

LIGHT MY FIRE!

In 2014, the *Wall Street Journal* (yes, the *Wall Street Journal*!) produced a three-minute instructional video of me demonstrating my time-tested toothpick technique for firing up my pipe. Be assured that I have no financial interests in the candle or toothpick industries. I recommend the technique solely on its merits. You can view my live demo on *YouTube* at https://youtu.be/2Zp1DoxodW0.

Chapter Three

Joints

Taking an Active Role with Rolling Paper

Ever since the marijuana renaissance of the 1960s, the joint has been hailed as the cannabis classic. Even classics wane in popularity and do not reign forever. Presently, only half of all cannabis smokers still smoke joints.[1] The rest have migrated to hand pipes, water pipes, and herbal vaporizers. Pass that joint? Instead, the time may have come to pass *on* that joint.

LET'S GET ROLLING

Grind or crumble some cannabis bud, spread the shreds or crumbs onto a thin sheet of slightly translucent paper, shape that sheet into a long and narrow cylinder, and then seal that cylindrical bundle along its length. You've now rolled yourself what decades ago was called a "reefer." Nowadays, one of the few vestiges of that nickname remains in references to the cult classic movie, *Reefer Madness*. The street slang name now more in vogue is "joint."

Simple and small, the joint is traditional, portable, concealable, disposable, and shareable. One convenient thing more—it is smokable. While it takes some practice to learn the science and fine art of rolling your own joint, once you've mastered the technique you can claim your cred as a cannabis connoisseur. If you're not there yet and in need of a tutorial to learn how to take an active role with rolling paper, you'll find an overabundance of instructional videos on YouTube. When less than five minutes in length, some videos are even cleverly edited precisely to 4' 20", the underground code number for cannabis. "Wanna hang out to toke up? Meet ya at 4:20 p.m."

CUTTING CORNERS IN YOUR USE OF ROLLING PAPERS

If you happen to have a pack of rolling papers stashed along with your stash, go dig it out and hold it in your hand. Do you really want to hold that paper in your lungs? Even thin paper merely adds to the toxic load, so the goal while rolling a joint is to use as little paper as possible.

Two thin joints, compared to one thick one, require two sheets of rolling paper rather than one sheet. That's one valid reason for rolling thick joints. With practice, regardless of how thick or thin the joint, one sheet should get you rolling, thus reducing your use of rolling paper.

Another way to cut corners in your use of rolling papers is to cut its corners. The inner edge of the paper that faces you when you begin to roll does not need to be as wide as the other edge farther away from you that has adhesive to seal the joint. So trim the two corners facing you where you start rolling. Some brands even omit that one extra step by providing two corners that already are trimmed.

The thinner the joint, the more room to breathe. Being cooled by air along all of its outer edges, joints aerate the smoke before it reaches your lips. That's why smoke from joints goes down the hatch more smoothly than smoke from most hand pipes. And that's why novices have an easier time first smoking joints than first smoking pipes. Indeed, for novices, joints may be the ideal "cannabinoid drug delivery system," but only for budding novices.

"Feds Go to Pot!" exclaimed the *New York Post*'s front-page headline when the Institute of Medicine (IOM) published its groundbreaking study about medicinal marijuana in 1999.[2] The study surprised proponents of the herbal remedy for both its accuracy and its advocacy. The IOM, however, cautioned that "[a]s a cannabinoid drug delivery system, marijuana cigarettes are not ideal."[3] Indeed, if you're no longer a tenderfoot and are already a master roller, then the time may have come to shed that skill and leave joints behind you.

THROUGH THICK AND THIN

Rolling papers are made from a variety of sources, the most common being wood pulp, which is so versatile that it is also used to make newsprint, book pages, writing paper, paper towels, and lest we forget, toilet paper. If a brand of rolling papers refrains from boasting about its contents, it's likely wood pulp. Other traditional fibers for rolling paper include sisal, rice straw, wheat straw, esparto, and flax. Outside of the United States, flax is called "linseed," while fabric and papers made from the fibrous stalk of the flax plant are called "linen." Esparto is a grass, so all the more appropriate for rolling "grass."

Some rolling papers claim the moral high ground by being made from ingredients that are all organically grown (OG). On the opposite spectrum of OG, others are bleached or dyed or carbonated. Some are sweetened with added flavors that, in order to pack a punch into a tiny sheet of thin paper, are mostly synthetic. Colored and flavored papers should be avoided as they are made with food additives that might be considered safe to eat but that have never been tested to be safe to combust and then to inhale. As a further effrontery, flavored papers detract from the savored taste of cannabis.

When bleached, papers retain chlorine residue.[4] When its fumes are inhaled, liquid chlorine bleach is so toxic that one whiff will make your head spin. No telling what some miniscule residue can do when combusted and inhaled. While some papers explicitly state that they are unbleached, many white-color papers are dead silent about it. During production, chemicals may be added to make the paper lighter, stronger, or longer burning. Some papers may also contain potassium nitrate to standardize the burn rate. That nitrate is as scary as it sounds and is linked to acute oral and respiratory irritation and damage.[5]

Different papers can affect the finished joint in terms of taste, burn rate, and drying effect on the mouth and throat. From among the vast array of brands in the marketplace, you would be wise to seek a paper that is free of additives such as bleach, dyes, and sweets. While all papers originate from plants and so are likely to be all vegan, some brands brazenly advertise "vegan" as a marketing ploy. Further, all glues are vegetable-based, usually comprising gum arabic, an adhesive that is made from the sap of the acacia tree. Despite the near universal use of vegetable-based gums, one brand tries to stand out by advertising in oversized capitalized letters "Vegan Gum." Assured of the plant-based nature of papers and glues, vegans can toke up with a sigh of relief.

Placed side by side, some papers look and feel thick, others thin. Perhaps alluding to an alluring phrase from condoms, some even advertise themselves as "ultra-thin." Traditional rice rolling papers are usually the thinnest, whereas hip hemp often stands out as the thickest. Rice papers, in part because they are thin, affect the taste of the cannabis the least. But let's be honest. By your third toke, both your taste buds and olfactory nerves are numbed by the smoke. After that, you can't discern much about the taste and smell of any joint.

ALL MIXED UP

Long-term numbed tongues and numbed noses are hallmarks of tobacco smoking. Two variations of the joint include the spliff and the blunt. The spliff, more common in Europe than in North America, mixes tobacco into the buzz. The blunt is cannabis rolled in a cigar wrapper made from ground tobacco and whole tobacco leaf. Spliffs and blunts are smoked primarily by tobacco users who seek to feed two habits with one stone.

When they mix tobacco with cannabis, tobacco smokers typically end up consuming up to 50 percent more cannabis in their blunts than when they smoke only cannabis in joints.[6] That's a waste of both cannabis and of lungs. Even worse, the joint venture of smoking tobacco together with cannabis increases the risk of developing both a tobacco habit and a cannabis habit.[7] As it omits the hook of tobacco that spliffs and blunts dangle in front of your nose, the joint is by far the safest of the three. Stated another way, though both present health risks, cannabis is safer than tobacco. We all already took this for granted.

HEMP FOR HIGH ROLLERS

Spurred largely from the burgeoning commerce in cannabis, an innovative fiber for rolling paper is hemp. Hemp and flax are the two toughest kids on the block. Hemp had been legally grown outside of the United States long before latecomer Americans relegalized its cultivation in

2018. Until then, hemp was legally imported, so hemp rolling papers were already being sold stateside for twenty years before its cultivation domestically.

You must be skillful to roll a joint with thin rice papers, whereas thick hemp papers make rolling easier for novices. As its identical twin, hemp makes botanical sense as the most compatible fiber for smoking cannabis. Yet, hip hemp paper does not add to any medicinal or psychoactive effects. To its credit, hemp paper rarely is bleached, while rice paper often is. You'd think that hemp would be the winner roller for all high rollers—but not so fast.

Rolling papers both hold the cannabis and hold back its combustion. (Think of them as likened to a car's fuel tank and a car's fuel injector.) Untreated rolling papers for tobacco can be classified into two main types. Slow burning and free burning. Slow burners snuff out if not puffed on persistently. Free burners, once lit, continue to burn without requiring a lot of huffing and puffing. Tobacco is itself chemically treated to burn continuously and freely.[8] Compared to tobacco, cannabis tends to burn slowly. Thus, cannabis in slow-burning paper burns slower still. When not puffed on constantly, such a joint snuffs out easily, requiring a second ignition. Unless you are holding the joint at arm's length or are using a flameless lighter, any potentially toxic second ignition is one too many.

Hemp papers are less porous than, say, rice, so hemp papers are slow burners. Hemp may be fashionable, but unless it is very thin it can prove impractical. When first introduced into the marketplace during the 1990s, hemp rolling papers were thick slow burners that snuffed out way too easily, so they garnered a bad reputation. Since then, they have been manufactured thinner and so are faster burners. Still, for rolling papers, wood pulp and rice and cotton remain the more dependable burners.

THE JOINT EFFECTS OF
PESTICIDES AND HEAVY METALS

While some questionable ingredients are intentionally added in, still others get inadvertently left in. Regulations setting limits on the use of pesticides on food plants do not apply to plants grown for their fibers to be made into textiles. For such fibrous plants, the sky's the limit. And the soil is the dumping ground. For instance, when grown on fields where cotton was previously rotated as a crop, due to residue of pesticides and herbicides in the soil, conventionally grown peanuts contain dangerously high levels of arsenic. This is worth your consideration if you partake of that cotton in the form of rolling papers.

When was the last time you noticed someone smoking a hand-rolled tobacco cig? Nowadays only a small fraction of papers sold directly to consumers are rolled into homemade tobacco cigarettes. Unless some of the remaining percentage is being used as mini toilet paper, it is no flight of imagination to conclude that the rest gets rolled into cannabis joints. For new product lines of rolling papers, the U.S. Food and Drug Administration (FDA) requires that companies offer samples, provide summaries of the results of any testing, and disclose a list of ingredients.[9] While the FDA sets regulatory standards for additives to tobacco, it sets no specific standards for what the actual ingredients in rolling papers should or should not be.

Organic tobacco is a niche market that has attracted few smokers. Unlike organic tobacco, demand for organic cannabis has grown steadily. Accordingly, lab tests have evolved to measure its purity. Yet, the same protocols of lab testing have rarely been applied to rolling papers. In 2020, in the first broad survey of its kind, Science of Cannabis Laboratories (SC Labs) performed random testing on seventy different rolling papers and twenty blunt wraps that were for sale online nationally and in the marketplace local to Santa Cruz, California.[10] In tests for pesticides and heavy metals, the blunt wraps predictably fared the worst because blunt wraps are made from tobacco. Let's skip the tobacco, so let's skip the blunt wraps.

While only two brands of rolling papers showed test results beyond the pesticide limits allowed by California for cannabis products, fifty-eight exceeded the heavy metal limits, most of them failing for traces of lead.[11] When digested in food or water and then deposited in the human body, lead causes brain damage and neurological disorders. When combusted as smoke and inhaled into the lungs, there's no telling what damage it inflicts. "Heavy metal" is also a subgenre of rock music. That music need not be a funeral march.

Health Tip for Choosing Papers: Until rolling papers are regulated and tested in the same way as are food and drink, it is prudent to be as conscious of the quality of the rolling paper as you are of the cannabis that you roll into them. When given the choice, seek rolling papers that are unbleached, unflavored, and made from fibers that are organically grown.

THE UNFILTERED TRUTH ABOUT FILTER TIPS

The cannabis in the butt end, in the vernacular called the "roach," serves to filter out tars streaming from the ember end. So far so good. But such good news turns bad when eventually you smoke down the roach for all that it's worth. You can keep your roaches large, and then just not keep them. If you discard them, you're making that tossed cannabis into a very costly filter. For a more economical filter, try filter tips.

Initially, filter tips found in tobacco cigarettes were made of cotton, which was a good thing. But that cotton was soaked in lye, which was a bad thing. Lye, also called sodium hydroxide, irritates and burns human skin. Obviously, such filter tips were not safe to stick into anyone's mouth. Later, filters were made of asbestos, until asbestos inhaled into the lungs was itself proven to cause cancer. Filter tips have had as bad a track record as the tobacco they were filtering and supposed to be rendering less harmful. Nowadays in the United States, only 1 percent of cigarette filters are made of charcoal,[12] while around 98 percent are made of cellulose acetate.[13]

Don't let the word "cellulose" fool you. Cellulose acetate is a cheap plastic derivative. The pliable base of analog motion picture and photographic film, too, is made of cellulose acetate. Film libraries often harbor a lingering odor from the outgassing of all the aging acetate. Just a few whiffs can cause headaches, both literally and figuratively. And never mind that the filter-tip cigarette butts consist of thousands of tiny microfibers that become the number-one plastic litter and toxic waste mindlessly thrown away into the environment.[14] The *away* that is away from the smokers is cast *toward* us tobacco nonsmokers and *toward* the already over-polluted environment.

In response to early studies linking lung cancer to smoking, the tobacco industry responded by inventing filter tips,[15] mere window dressings, so that their customers could delude themselves into believing that the windows behind the curtains were not filled with soot and grime. Studies have shown that cellulose-acetate filter tips do not effectively reduce the incidence of lung cancer from tobacco cigarettes. Rather, they only postpone the cancer from developing by five years, and they shift the cancer from one type to another type.[16] One reason is that, cigarette for cigarette, a filter-tip cig contains less tobacco than a cig with none.[17] Smoking less tobacco postpones cancer, but does not banish it. Postponement is not prevention, while cancer is cancer, and death is death.

Cigarette filters indeed do effectively trap some of the tar and ash in tobacco smoke, so they do safeguard against the health hazards of that gunk that was trapped. But that trapped gunk is hardly worth singing about because nicotine also gets trapped. To compensate for lost nicotine, many smokers smoke more cigarettes, and therefore more tobacco, and therefore still more gunk, just not the gunk trapped in the tip.

Filter tips primarily provide only a psychologically comforting placebo effect, proven ultimately useless by the hundreds of thousands of tobacco smokers of filter-tip cigarettes who every year still die of lung cancer and other respiratory diseases. Filter tips are money makers for cigarette makers for two reasons. Any given length of a filter tip costs less than the same volume stuffed with tobacco. And a filter tip offers smokers the false assurance that they can continue to smoke and therefore will continue to buy the cigarette makers' cigarettes. Continue to smoke, they do, until their last dying breath.

BURNING QUESTIONS ABOUT
FILTER TIPS FOR CANNABIS

The Institute for Cancer Prevention formerly had been called the American Health Foundation. Before 2004, when the institute went bankrupt and disappeared in a puff of smoke, its researchers had devoted much resources to study the effects of filter tips on cigarettes. Those researchers offered the opinion that tobacco filters would prove ineffective for cannabis because, if applied to joints, whatever filter that trapped tar inadvertently would also filter out cannabinoids.[18] The researchers did not offer any further advice, effectively leaving cannabis smokers in the lurch.

If we are to reach any conclusions, it would be that to compensate for lost cannabinoids trapped by filter tips, we cannabis smokers would end up smoking more. Thus, we would cancel out any slim benefit of a filter tip made of cellulose acetate. If you examine this duality closely, you'll realize tar and cannabinoids exist in unison. Blocking one only comes at the expense of blocking the other.

As alternatives to cellulose acetate, filter tips made solely of all cotton, all wool, or all hemp do exist on the marketplace. Applied to cannabis joints, they indeed should trap tar and ash, but they lack scientific testing for effectiveness in not also blocking cannabinoids. Corn husk or charcoal filter tips originally intended for tobacco are sometimes promoted by marketers as suitable for use with cannabis. Suitable, sure. Desirable, maybe. Proven, not. Their claims are unsubstantiated by any documentation or lab tests proving that such filter tips do not remove cannabinoids. Nor are there any studies that have studied the lack of their studies. With no regulatory oversight to reign in those claims, anything goes and anything gets said.

Tar and ash are not the only harmful constituents in smoke, be it of tobacco or of cannabis. Noxious gases also lurk within and emanate out. In theory, a filter that increases the oxygen content in smoke could convert the carbon monoxide in smoke into harmless carbon dioxide. Until such a carbon monoxide filter is perfected, that remains only an untested theory, and like any theory it is one that could lead to a dead end.

Canada is a nation a decade ahead of the United States in regard to drug law reform on the federal level. Until recently, Canada was home to the largest cannabis corporation in the world. In 2020, that botanical baton was passed on to a leviathan corporation in the United States. Until cannabis is legalized nationwide, research by the cannabis industry has been slow. The cannabis industry has directed research to alternatives to smoking but not to improvements in safer smoking. A filter tip to remove the noxious fumes, the tar, and the ash from cannabis smoke without also removing cannabinoids just might be under development and under wraps in a lab somewhere. Maybe there's some ongoing research and development that might prove to be just what we've been waiting for. But while waiting, don't hold your breath.

Health Tip about Filter Tips: Once you have filtered out all the hype about filter tips, you will come to understand that none has yet been proven effective for cannabis. Until then, don't waste your money. Don't waste your breath.

TIPS ABOUT SMOKING TIPS

Smoking tips, also called crutches, indeed are worth your devoting your breath to them. While the ambulatory accessories called crutches usually are used in pairs, the smoking crutch is used singly. To avoid offending the disability community, we'll stick with the phrase "smoking tips." Smoking tips are popular in Europe but something of a novelty in the United States. While smoking tips are commercially available under the misnomer "filter tips," you can make your own.

Start with strips of paperboard or heavy stock paper such as from file cards or business cards. Or start with thin non-corrugated cardboard, which can be found in the outer packaging for near-at-hand rolling papers or matchbooks. Trim a piece to the width of a typical cigarette filter and to a length three or four times its width. Next roll it into a coil, as though shaping sushi or a tortilla wrap. Apply pressure with your fingertips to retain the smoking tip's coil shape. Moistening it with the tip of your tongue can help to keep it coiled. Or add a dab of nontoxic glue stick. Before rolling, place the coil into the rolling paper at the end that will serve as your mouthpiece. If your tip is long enough, allow some of it to stick out from the rolling paper. Add your cannabis along the remainder of the paper. Then get rolling.

The coiled smoking tip might trap a wee bit of tar and ash, but that is only secondary, because some cannabinoids would get trapped in that tar. A smoking tip serves other useful purposes. Some smokers who drool on the tip of the joint may cause the tip to collapse, blocking air flow, and thus slackening the draw. The smoking tip keeps the tip open and air flow unimpeded.

By reducing waste, the coiled smoking tip also serves as a clear cost saver. It prevents raw cannabis from flowing out the end and into your mouth. It also replaces the role of a leftover roach that you might trash when done, thus sparing you from intentionally discarding any cannabis. Perish the thought of following the example of tobacco smokers by mindlessly casting your roach into the environment.

Paper drinking straws cut into small segments provide an alternative to coiled smoking tips. Until recently, paper straws had been a specialty item usually relegated to health food stores. With the rise of our post-plastic conscientious consumer ethic, paper straws have made a comeback in supermarkets. So seek a straw made of paper rather than plastic just in case you burn your joint right down to the smoking tip and unwittingly burn the tip too. When rolling the joint, you might need to apply a tiny dab of nontoxic glue stick to prevent the straw from slipping out of the joint. Cutting longer segments allows you to extend the tip past the rolling paper, making it all the more protective against burns.

The most important feature of both coiled and straw smoking tips is burn prevention. Just as most joints start out narrower and smaller than tobacco cigarettes, most roaches end up shorter than cigarette butts. The burning ember of cannabis then dangles perilously close to your tongue, your lips, and your fingertips. With the addition of a smoking tip, the burning roach won't scorch any fragile part of your body. Burns, after all, are not conducive to good health.

Health and Safety Tips about Smoking Tips: Smoking tips offer three benefits. They reduce waste and therefore save you money. They prevent the tip of the joint from collapsing and therefore assure air flow. And, most importantly, they create a safe distance to buffer between you and the burning embers and so are safeguards against burns.

ROACH CLIPS AND CIGARETTE HOLDERS

Variations of smoking tips that you neither insert into nor discard with each joint include roach clips and cigarette holders.

Roach clips originally were devised from alligator clips used by electricians and locking forceps used by surgeons. Rather than hold the roach, you hold the clip that holds the roach. In a pinch, you can improvise one by tearing a matchbook cover free from its matches and holding the roach between the fold of the cover. Now sold at most smoke shops, roach clips are simple devices that can come embellished with psychedelic colors or funky logos. Roach clips safeguard against burns and stains on your fingertips. But still some danger lurks for stains and burns on your lips and tongue.

Cigarette holders are long, slender tubes similar to pipe stems. Like pipe stems, they are made of plastic, ceramic, or wood, while some luxury items akin to jewelry are made of silver. Like straws when used for making smoking tips and same as pipes, holders provide a safe distance between you and the joint's burning embers. You will not burn or stain your fingertips, lips, or tongue. Less smoke will get in your eyes, making them less bloodshot. Less smoke will permeate your hair and clothing, preventing them from smelling stale. If you daydream and let ashes drop, they will less likely fall on you or your clothing, preventing them from smelling stinky.

Inserting your joint into a holder is like holding up your pants with both suspenders and a belt. If the rolling paper serves as suspenders and the cigarette holder as belt, you might as well skip the suspenders. You might as well smoke a pipe.

Safety Tip about Cigarette Holders: Rather than resort to a cigarette holder, you might as well skip the troublesome and risky rolling paper altogether and use only a pipe.

A NEW TAKE ON TOKES

Let's say that you're holding your expertly rolled joint, have near at hand a roach clip for when you'll need it, and are now ready to toke. How to toke that joint? When smoking, be aware that half of the smoke, and therefore the cannabinoids, is lost to side stream, which is the smoke that never reaches your mouth. Between tokes, much smoke is lost at the burning end and through aeration along the sides of the paper. In contrast, with hand pipes and water pipes, there is no aeration because there is no paper, and you can always cap the bowl in between tokes. When smoking joints, how then to most efficiently make use of the little smoke that does reach your mouth? Long pulls or short? Between pulls, long breaks or short? Questions, questions, troubling our minds—and troubling our lungs.

Leave it to the Dutch to blaze a trail where American cannabis corporations have yet to tread. In the United States, recreational and medicinal cannabis corporations seldom fund research. In contrast, the Netherlands' largest medicinal cannabis corporation, Bedrocan, either sponsors extensive independent research or provides for free the cannabis used in that research.[19]

A Dutch study published in 2008 addressed how precisely to best keep that joint burning so that you can squeeze it for all the THC that it's worth.[20] As you'd expect, the study found that longer pulls introduced more THC into the blood. Similarly, more frequent pulls of once every fifteen seconds compared to once every thirty or sixty seconds raised the temperature of the burning joint, which in turn introduced more THC into the blood. But there's a catch that was overlooked by the researchers. As mentioned earlier in this chapter, tars and cannabinoids exist in unison. Higher temperatures also introduce more tar, more carbon monoxide, and other noxious fumes into the lungs.

Staying conscientious and keeping count of how deeply or how frequently you take a drag can quickly become a drag in the colloquial sense, too. All the better if you lose count. The act of smoking should be enjoyable and leisurely, otherwise why bother? Another way to rev up the joint to its hottest without having to keep puffing away and to keep count is to invite your friends to help out.

INSIDE OF A SMALL CIRCLE OF FRIENDS

Cannabis is often partaken as a communal experience, even as a ritual. In the same way that alcohol works as a social icebreaker, cannabis can serve as a stimulant to conversation, sometimes intimate and meaningful, others times merely zany and foolish. The act of sharing a smoke can forge a bond among strangers, can deepen a bond among friends, can spread joy throughout the land, and can spread disease throughout the household.

In 1988, a friend and I were invited by Bob Marley's mother, Cedella Booker, to visit her in her home in Miami. As a gracious host and as the mother of the spirit of Rastafari incarnate, Ms. Booker ritually shared some holy herb with us—but with a twist. No lit joint was passed around. Rather, she bestowed upon each of us our own personal joints. Only the matches were passed around. This shattering of cannabis convention at that time was a revelation to me. Whether she did not want others to share their cooties with her, or she did not want to share her cooties with others, a joint of one's own made perfect sense from the perspective of oral hygiene. Alternatively, she could have more closely observed tradition by providing each of us with a cigarette holder, and then we could have passed around a single joint. Afterwards, though, those holders would have required retrieving and sanitizing. Easier to provide each of us with our own personal joints.

Let's not forget that the last step in rolling a joint is sealing it. That requires moistening the narrow strip of adhesive along its edge. You should use a cotton swab moistened with water. Yet most people lick it with their tongues, meaning with their saliva. While most of that saliva gets burned with the joint, the saliva on the roach end in your mouth does not. No matter how much care you both might take not to drool on the roach end of a joint that you shared, you might as well be kissing your friend who rolled it.

When pipes, water pipes, herbal vaporizers, and especially joints routinely get passed around, that's fine if it's with your lover with whom you may already be sharing hugs and kisses and so much more. But it is prudent to avoid sharing bodily fluids with mere casual acquaintances. At dinner, if you share a bottle of wine with your intimate dinner date, the two of you do not drink out of the same glass. You may share the bottle, but you do not share the glass. In the same spirit in our post-pandemic society, do *not* pass that joint.

Chapter Four

Hand Pipes

More Than Just a Pipe Dream

Rolling papers first rolled onto the scene in the sixteenth century. Until then, when people intentionally inhaled burning herbs, they sniffed them ambiently, like sage in a sweat lodge, or they smoked them directly, like pot in a pipe. Pipes sculpted from stone have been unearthed in archaeological digs throughout the world, some dating as far back into the misty past as six millennia ago. In our present Stoned Age, pipe-smoking traditionalists can take comfort knowing that they are reenacting ancient rituals first practiced by our prehistoric ancestors.

PUT THIS IN YOUR PIPE AND SMOKE IT

The act of smoking a pipe provides several advantages over smoking a joint, including enabling you to be less hurried, less wasteful, less toxic, and less irritating to your respiratory tract.

Less Hurried: Different herbs combust at differing rates. When smoked leisurely in a pipe, tobacco leaves tend to stay lit, while cannabis flowers easily extinguish. That's not necessarily a bad thing. By snuffing out between tokes, that allows you to sit back and relax and take your sweet time. Time for what? Time to think heavenly thoughts, to ponder your daydreams, and to conjure up a few pipedreams.

To solve problems, the 1930s cartoon character Grampy, granddad of Betty Boop, used to put on his thinking cap. When he hit upon a solution, the light bulb in his cap would light up. In real life, we smok-ers can light up our thinking pipes.

Less Wasteful: Once you light up a joint, you tend to rush the act of smoking, continuing until you've reduced the joint down to a roach whether or not you really need any more of the rest of that joint. While you are exhaling or daydreaming or philosophizing with your smoking companion, the joint continues burning, so the smoke that is lost to side stream is wasted. In contrast, with a pipe in between puffs you can cap the bowl to prevent smoke from escaping into thin air, thus conserving your precious and usually costly cannabis. This holds especially true if your smoking session is solo rather than social.

According to one estimate, a pipe transfers 40 to 50 percent of the cannabinoids in cannabis, while a joint relays to your mouth only 10 to 20 percent.[1] Expressed in terms of THC alone, up to half is lost to side stream in a joint.[2] Thus a pipe can be two to four times more cost efficient. A precise calculation of the cost savings is possible only with laboratory analysis of the cannabinoid level in your blood. Lacking a nearby lab, I estimate that to reach the same degree of medication or same level of euphoria, I need less than half the amount of cannabis when stuffing a pipe than when rolling a joint. Expressed as an automo-tive metaphor, to drive to Nirvana in a joint, I need two fill-ups, while in a pipe I need only one tankful of the same octane gasoline. Your own mileage will vary.

The choice is not between getting twice as high or medicated once or getting half as high or medicated twice. Rather, it is between consuming the same portion of cannabis in one session or spreading it out into two. Smoke one pipeful, and get one free.

Less Toxic: While pipes also happen to spare you the slightly extra cost of rolling papers, more importantly they spare your lungs the extra risk of extra smoke from burning papers. That added smoke might be warranted if the papers were medicinal or psychoactive, but papers do not contribute to any relief or any high. No, not even rolling papers made from hemp contribute, as hemp paper is derived from the fibrous stalk rather than from the cannabinoid-rich flower.

As discussed in detail in chapter 2, a less toxic load applies here only if great care is taken when reigniting the bowl. Matches or butane lighters do not pass muster. Caution is more effectively exercised with toothpicks lit from candles or with flameless lighters.

Less Irritating: Pipes provide another respiratory benefit that joints otherwise lack. Smoke is hot and dry, which dries out your mouth and throat. By absorbing the heat, a pipe's stem cools down the smoke before you take a hit.[3] The longer the pipe stem, the cooler the smoke. That is way cool.

Think of historic ads for mentholated cigarettes that promoted the false promise of silky-smooth smoke. Without causing any actual decrease of temperature, synthetic menthol merely numbed the tongue and throat. There's no need for the ruse of mistaken sensations when you smoke from a pipe with a long stem that really does lower the heat. Consider a stem to be long when it is at least the length of your two fingers.

THE STEM: THE TUNNEL AT THE END OF THE LIGHT

Accustomed to feeling irritation in their throats and lungs when smoking, first-time long-stem pipe smokers who don't feel anything going down their hatches tend to take very long and very big hits. Filling their lungs to the point of bursting, novices then gag and explode into a coughing fit. Such gagging is the lungs' way of sounding an alarm. Hello, brain, are you listening?

Pipes provide still one more form of respiratory relief. Pipes trap tars that condensate along the inner walls of their stems, also called their shanks. Tars are mistaken by some tenderfoot smokers as cannabinoid-rich resins. Make no mistake, those are not products of the resinous glands of the cannabis flower, rather they are tars, and tars are toxic hydrocarbons released during burning.

We know that tars and cannabinoids are trapped in unison in joints in the roach end, and if filter tips are used, by the filters, too.[4] And we know that tars and cannabinoids are trapped in unison in the water of water pipes.[5] In the absence of any scientific study to cite, we do not know for sure but we can speculate that some cannabinoids are trapped by the tars that condensate along the inner walls of pipe stems. If so, is there a way to minimize the amount of cannabinoids that are trapped? Perhaps there is.

Compared to cannabinoid-infused smoke, particulates probably are heavier, and tars and ash are particulates. When you smoke, you should obey the laws of gravity and apply them to your advantage. Elevate the mouthpiece of the pipe above the level of the bowl. That way when tar adheres to the inner walls of the stem, that sticky tar will in turn capture some ash. The longer the stem, the more the tar and ash can potentially stick to the walls with less gooey tar and bulky ash making their way to your mouthpiece and to you. In theory, the lighter-weight cannabinoids would only minimally be trapped by tar, so most cannabinoids would successfully reach their destination, namely you.

A pipe whose stem is arm's length is long enough for anyone to handle. Smoke shops sometimes go to great lengths to stock long-stemmed pipes that mimic American Indian peace pipes, often with faux eagle feathers dangling from them. These are merely novelty items, suitable only for displaying as wall decorations. After multiple uses, the long stems would get clogged with tar and ash, but you would be unable to access the central area of the stems to clean them. Stuffed pipes would turn into ornamental conversation pieces, including you talking about how you wish you could clean them to continue to use them. So skip the American Indian peace pipe, and look to England.

The British term for a long-stemmed pipe whose bowl is made of wood or clay is the "churchwarden pipe." Having been popularized in book and film by the *Hobbit* trilogy, they have recently been nicknamed "Hobbit pipes." When purchasing one, be sure to buy the pipe cleaners sold with them that exceed or at least match the length of the stem. The German term for a long-stemmed wooden pipe is translated as a "reading pipe" because the long stem allows readers to look down at a book without the smoke getting in their eyes. Even when not multitasking by reading a book while smoking, you will reap benefits by smoking with a pipe with a long stem.

DIVIDE AND CONQUER

Very long stems should be segmented for easy cleaning and for convenient storage. You can piece together long stems from several metal segments sold piecemeal by most smoke shops. But metal parts impart an unpleasant tinny aftertaste to the smoke, and they are heavy and cumbersome to lug. Wood, a natural fiber, is lightweight and imparts either a more agreeable aroma or none at all.

Despite a diversity of pipes sold in the marketplace, segmented long-stemmed wooden pipes are rarities. Asian Indian import stores sometimes stock them, but such stores are located only in the very largest cities. You might need to conduct an extensive search for such a pipe, but your search will be worth it. For a peek at this author demonstrating his twenty-five-year-old segmented long-stemmed wooden pipe, view a three-minute instructional video produced in 2014 by the *Wall Street Journal*: https://youtu.be/2Zp1DoxodW0.

In the absence of long-stemmed pipes in smoke shops, you might try performing some musical improvisations. Try a toy store and look for an inexpensive wooden flute intended as a starter instrument for the kiddies. The narrower its air canal, the better, as some can be too wide. Tape closed its finger holes, affix a pipe bowl at the far end, and presto, you now have one long-stemmed stealth wooden pipe.

In the olden days of total prohibition, stealth pipes abounded that were fashioned to look like stubby cigars that never burned down to a stub, or like lipsticks that never adorned a lip, or like felt markers that never made a mark. Some smoke shops presently sell decoy drumsticks that never beat a drum. The drumstick is sawed in half crosswise and then hollowed out lengthwise. A socket is whittled on one end of each half so that the two halves can be joined together or taken apart. When joined together with a bowl inserted on one end, they can attune you to the sound of a different drummer.

PASS UP THE PEACE PIPE

Note that when you engage in the unhygienic act of gathering into a cannabis circle with friends to pass the peace pipe, your joint, or your vaporizer, if someone slobbers about it, they will also be sharing their bacteria and viruses that can transmit a host of contagious respiratory diseases. Thus the otherwise honorable notion of sharing must be practiced with caution. At the tip of the stem, the mouthpiece marks the intimate meeting place between you and your drug paraphernalia.

A manufacturer that markets its own interchangeable mouthpiece claims that its testing has shown that the mouthpiece of the average pot pipe harbors more bacteria than a public toilet seat. While that comparison would be fitting for a public pot pipe, the last time I have seen one of those was in 1988 at a regional Rainbow Gathering. In our post-pandemic society, you could provide each of your cannabis companions with a baby bottle nipple to insert into the mouthpiece of your pipe. Yet just as condoms can detract from the joys of lovemaking, so would modified pacifiers detract from smoking.

Instead, distribute the segments of your segmented long-stem pipe among your small circle of friends, then pass around the last segment with the bowl. Everyone shares the same bowl, but puff from their individual segments applied to the communal bowl when it comes their way. Think of octopus-like hookahs with one single bowl but several tubular stems.

Pipe stems are made of wood, glass, stone, silicone, acrylic, ceramic, or metal. When stems are short, non-wooden pipes can get too hot to handle. Take care with metal stems as they are especially efficient at conducting heat that can burn your fingertips and lips. Pipes made solely of borosilicate glass, often embedded with psychedelic colors, are less prone than other forms of glass to crack when heated, though more prone to break or shatter if dropped. Either way, cuts from glass shards are not conducive to good health.

THE BOWL: THE ROSE BOWL, THE SUGAR BOWL, THE CANNABIS BOWL

While wood is ideal for stems, it poses a problem initially for use as bowls. Brand new wooden bowls can burn ever so slightly, hence the aroma some lend to the cannabis smoke. Wood thus requires an initiation ceremony in which an empty bowl is puffed upon but not inhaled. Because where there's fire, there's smoke.

Wooden bowls made of hardwood, once initiated, will hardly scorch again because they require higher temperatures to ignite than does the cannabis flower. In North America, wooden bowls are usually hand carved or machine carved from native hardwoods such as oak, maple, beech, or walnut. Some visually appealing pipes are carved from cherrywood with slivers of cherry tree bark still attached. Briarwood, imported from Europe and Africa, is the most heat-resistant of all woods and so is favored for wooden pipes intended for tobacco. But tobacco bowls are too big for cannabis.

Corncob pipes tend to have smaller bowls, but they ignite way too easily. Its outer shell, sometimes varnished with shellac, is especially flammable and can ignite along the rim of the bowl. The most hazardous are the tiny, cheap pipes displayed overhead on convenience store pegboards. While corncob's low cost lends itself to throwaway single use when you travel, its first use poses danger.

Metal bowls, even when too hot to handle, do remain non-flammable. Smoke shops sell them piecemeal the same as metal stems, so metal bowls can be accessorized onto wooden stems.

Turkish meerschaum and ceramic are the safest bowls.

Soapstone and sandstone pipes are sculpted as bowls and stems both in one small piece, but their stems are too short for safe use.

Glass hand pipes, distinct from glass water pipes, also have bowls and stems both in one piece, so their stems are usually too short and their bowls are always too hot to handle. But small glass pipes whose bowls become too hot to handle do provide one feature that can be used to an advantage. You can use them like a crack pipe. Rather than ignite the cannabis through the top of the bowl, you can heat the underside or sides of the bowl. By heating the cannabis rather than burning it, you effectively turn the small glass pipe into a primitive but pocket-size vaporizer. For more about vaporizers, see chapter 6. For more about crack pipes, see chapter 666.

Flat-bottomed bowls are features of most metal pipes that many other bowls lack. It's puzzling and annoying that many pipes that are marketed for smoking cannabis have rounded bottoms. You simply cannot place round-bottomed pipes steady upon a table with any confidence that the pipe will not flop over and spill the precious contents of the bowl. There ought to be a law banning pipes with rounded bottoms. No, wait! Most prohibitionist laws prove to be miserable failures. Just be vigilant to buy or piece together only pipes with level bottoms.

DIY: Consider constructing a hybrid of your own of a long but segmented wooden stem that ends at a small stone or ceramic bowl. The traditional Moroccan *sepsi*, with its long wooden but single-segment stem and small clay bowl, exemplifies this. Heads up, head shops! Are you listening?

THE APPLE OF MY EYE

In the absence of a local smoke shop or when you are in a pinch, you can always improvise a one-piece pipe on your own. A perennial favorite is the legendary apple of the Garden of Eden. The apple even adds a hint of moisture if not also a fruity flavor as you draw on it. As a bonus feature, many apples sit upright on a table. So be sure to select an apple with a level bottom.

DIY: Start at the top. Carve out an eyelet at the stem and continue down halfway into the core. Next, from the side, hollow out a second eyelet, also halfway into the core. The two tunnels should meet, forming an L-like shape. The stem top is your bowl. Insert a screen, and you're on your way. When you're done smoking, remove the screen, and eat the rest of the apple, which can replenish moisture to your parched mouth and throat. As smoking depletes the human body of vitamin C, an added bonus is that eating the apple will provide you with a bit of vitamin C, though not as much as when you compare apples with oranges.

SCREENING FOR DRUGS

The bowls of pipes intended for tobacco are larger than those designed for cannabis. To reduce the depth of the chamber of the bowl, you can insert a screen. Actually, even small bowls require a screen in order to block both bits of bud and specks of ash from reaching your mouth.

Avoid resorting to a makeshift screen from aluminum foil punctured with pinholes. After just one use, the foil corrodes. After a second use, it crumbles. By the third, it disintegrates as though into thin air. Where did it go? Into the smoke and into your lungs.

Instead, use screens made from more durable metals such as brass or steel. In a pinch, you can pilfer the screen found inside the housing of the nozzle of a sink faucet or shower head. But faucet screens often are dense and brittle, so it's better to purchase pliable ones from smoke shops. Theirs are smokescreens that do not disguise or conceal.

Smoke shops sell coin-shaped screens in various diameters and in meshes of various densities. U.S. ten-cent dime-sized screens fit most bowls, and five-cent nickel-sized fit the rest. If you need a still bigger size screen, then—unless you're sharing a buzz with a family of gorillas—your bowl is too big.

Some pipe screens are coated with a thin layer of plastic or wax applied to assure a grip to the punch press that cuts the circles out of the sheet of metal mesh. Stay safe by burning off that coating before inserting the screen into the bowl of your pipe. First toast it in the flame of a lighter or match or candle. If someone asks why are you toasting your screen, just answer that you are screening for drugs.

GOOD CLEAN FUN

To keep your drug pipeline flowing, replace that screen regularly. Oh sure, you can clean it the same way that you clean glass pipes and vaporizer parts, for instance by soaking the screen in isopropyl alcohol, also called rubbing alcohol. (See chapter 5 about water pipes for more about using iso alcohol.) But screens are so inexpensive and tiny that they are hardly worth fussing over. Besides, safely disposing of the sullied alcohol is way more hassle than trashing a screen.

Whenever you do replace the screen, also clean out the gunk from the rest of the pipe to prevent tar and ash from reaching the mouthpiece and then your mouth. If your pipe does become clogged, then you've waited too long. If convenient, after each smoking session take apart the bowl and the stem(s). Expel any loose ash by blowing into each chamber, as if you were a musician tooting your own horn. A sound check alone can inform you when it's time to replace the screen and to clean the bowl and stem(s). Do you hear a loud whoosh, or only a soft whimper, or barely a muffled gasp?

For preferred long stems with multiple segments, perform a visual check on each segment. Like a cliché pirate peering through a spyglass, peek into each segment to make sure you can see the light at the end of the tunnel. When needed, you usually need to clean only the one segment closest to the bowl. If the segment with the mouthpiece needs cleaning, then once again you've waited too late.

Cleaning can get messy, so spread a sheet of newspaper on your table to serve as a disposable tablecloth. Cleaning can also be a drudgery, but find joy in knowing that any gooey gunk on the table, on your cleaning tools, and on your hands is better there than in your lungs. If you loathe

the cleanup, stop griping and just stick with smoking joints. Here's how joints and pipes are similar. The same time you take after use to clean a pipe, you take before use to roll a joint. Yet here's how joints and pipes differ. The same gooey gunk you clean from a pipe, you suck into your lungs from a joint.

To clean out stems, bristle-coated wires appropriately called pipe cleaners are ideal drug paraphernalia. The standard length is six inches (15 cm). While still clean, pipe cleaners are also fun to play with, for instance, to twist into origami-like ornamental figures. Pipe cleaners for high-octane pipes are one foot (30 cm) long. Some long stems do not allow easy insertion of pipe cleaners, in which case bamboo skewers intended as cookware will do the job.

To scrape out bowls, sandwich picks that are twice the length and twice the width of toothpicks are useful. Also, blunt-tipped knives or disposable X-acto (Exacto) blades come in handy. Speaking of hands, to avoid soiling your hands with any gunk while cleaning, wear a pair of vinyl or nitrile exam gloves. When donning gloves, just remember that two lefts do not make a right.

ASHES TO ASHES, SMOKE TO SMOKE

All the aforementioned health tips about using pipes pale in comparison with heeding one simple last step in the smoking process. Do not smoke that bowlful down to just ash. Quit while you're a head—a pothead, that is. Otherwise, on that final toke, you risk inhaling mostly ash, but hardly any smoke. If you're left with little or no ash to clean out of the pipe bowl, where the heck did it all go? Dump that ash into an ashtray, not into your lungs.

Chapter Five

Water Pipes

The Big Bong Theory

First made of bamboo in Thailand, the water pipe had for centuries been traditionally used for tobacco. A distinct type of water pipe, the hookah of the Middle East, also moonlighted for hashish. In North America, smokers nowadays use water pipes primarily for cannabis. Some models are compact and portable, while most are designed for tabletops. Some models are made of silicone or ceramic, while most are made with bowls of glass or metal, and with bodies of fragile glass or durable acrylic. The two ingredients that all models share are cannabis and water.

ODE TO YOUTH

Glass bodies have morphed into ornate and sculptural designs whose creation has elevated the craft into an artform. Any dubious reputation that straight society may have cast upon this sculptural artform is due to their use almost exclusively for cannabis. In stoner lingo, the ornate tabletop model is cherished as a "bong," while the pocket-size model is nicknamed a "bubbler." When smoke shops sold bongs and bubblers during prohibition, they could endorse their use for tobacco only. Perhaps in whispers and under wraps, they called them "bongs." (Hush, hush.) When reverting to abiding by state laws and store policy, shopkeepers called them "water pipes." (Wink, wink.)

As accoutrements of cannabis culture, the bong and bubbler might evoke an image of a laidback teenager sporting a 420-logo embroidered on his backward-donned baseball cap or emblazoned on her rainbow-colored tie-dyed tee-shirt. As a teenager, you might have been one such starry-bloodshot-eyed stoner. Even if your parents were aging hippies who voiced tolerance of your youthful drug use, prudence may have dictated that you conceal your use and hide your stash anyway. Part of your hidden treasures probably included a pack of rolling papers or a pocket-sized pipe. Unless your bedroom or basement had drop-down ceilings, water pipes were too big and bulky to conceal, so its possession remained off limits to you. Upon leaving home and moving into your first pad or settling into your first-year college-student dorm room, your rite of passage may have included the purchase of your first bong—oops, of your first water pipe.

WATER PIPES ARE COOL

In addition to granting you bragging rights among your friends, your new bong enabled you to indulge in some late nights of serious smoking, because, oh joy, now you were being kind to your lungs. Just hearing the bubbling sound calmed your sense of mental well-being. And when you were done, pouring the chamber's clouded water down the drain comforted your state of physical health. When you smelled the stink, you were thankful that the stink was in your sink and not in your lungs. Gosh, you thought, that was stinky enough to make you never want to smoke again, or anyway never smoke with anything other than your trusty bong. With its use, you were certain you were doing your lungs a big favor by cooling and moistening the smoke—or so you believed.

Your assumptions were only partially correct. Yes, water pipes do cool the otherwise hot and scratchy smoke. But contrary to most young smokers' expectations, water pipes do not moisten it. Hot and dry, smoke desiccates and irritates your mouth and throat, which makes you more susceptible to colds and flu. The parched air of indoor heating, which dries out your nasal passage and mouth and throat, contributes to the higher incidence of such diseases in winter. To counteract the arid air, room humidifiers add water vapor into the air. While it is reassuring to consider water pipes as humidifiers for your mouth and throat, that analogy does not hold water.

Long-stemmed pipes, too, cool smoke without moistening it. But you don't expect a hand pipe to moisten the smoke because it contains no water. The power of suggestion is strong, especially to impressionable young minds. The bubbling water in the bong might have led you to believe that the smoke bubbles gather some moisture along the route from the small bowl to your big mouth. Yet, chemical analysis of the smoke exiting the water pipe has proven otherwise. The mere passage through water does not necessarily impart any steam into the smoke. You might be as high as a kite, but the smoke remains as dry as a bone.

ASHES TO ASHES, LUNG TO LUNG

Although smoke bubbles absorb no moisture from the water, the water does gather something from the smoke. For both cannabis and tobacco, the water purifies the smoke bubbles by trapping an appreciable amount of some water-soluble toxins including hydrogen cyanide, much of the hydrocarbons, and much of the particulate matter including tars and ash.[1]

Particulate matter is quite simply the solid minuscule particles in the air we breathe. The trick is to avoid inhaling them. In urban air, particulates include soot and the dust that you can see floating indoors in the air spotlighted by sunlight against a darkened background. Particulates also include sulphates and nitrates that you should be thankful that you don't see. In cannabis smoke, the particulate matter we both see and inhale is ash. There is no safe level of particulate matter in the lungs. Any level is harmful. If minuscule particulates penetrate deep within our lungs, they reach the alveoli, the air-filled sacs that exchange oxygen for carbon dioxide. In comes the good, out goes the bad—but not necessarily all of the bad. If ash were to slip past the cilia cells and enter the bloodstream, it would reach every part of the body, from head to toe, from brain cells to bone mass.

An alternative method of reducing your intake of ash is by smoking with a hand pipe and then *not* toking the cannabis down to its last few hits. If you call time-out at that end zone, you will avoid sucking in much ash. This would hardly be economical unless your cannabis were homegrown. But if you needed to be really frugal, you probably couldn't afford cannabis in the first place. Just as effective and more economical, you can avoid inhaling ash by smoking with a water pipe or by vaping with a vaporizer. (More about vaporizers in the next chapter.)

THE WATER THAT MAKES A PIPE A WATER PIPE

When you filled your water pipe straight from the faucet, you used lukewarm or cold water, right? Cold water cools the smoke, yes. Experienced water pipe users claim that hot water traps more tar.[2] If so, a dual-chambered water pipe would prove ideal, with the first chamber filled with hot water, and the second chamber with cold. While such models do exist, most water pipes are the single-chamber deal.

As most water pipes lack two chambers, you can resort to other health-promoting techniques. Change the water in the chamber midway through each smoking session. A vacuum cleaner loses efficiency as its dust bag fills up. It's the same for the water as it fills with stench.

Another effective health tip is to use non-chlorinated water. If you draw tap water from your sink's faucet, pass it through a filter. In the absence of a filter, allow the water to sit in an open container for twenty-four hours. The chlorine will evaporate. Think of an indoor swimming pool from whose locker room you can smell the disinfectant even from afar. That's the chlorine evaporating from the pool and into the ventilation system where it recirculates into the locker room. Emerge from a swim and, until you take a shower in even more diluted chlorinated water, the lingering antiseptic odor of chlorine will cling to your skin and hair all day long. Chlorine gas was used during gas warfare in the trenches of World War I. We already drink too much chlorinated water from municipal water systems, so avoid inhaling chlorine in smoke that's been filtered by the stuff.

In theory, chlorine bleach intended for removing laundry stains might be effective for cleaning stains in bongs. In practice, chlorine bleach is noxious to inhale, caustic to handle, and leaves a lingering antiseptic odor on your bong, its mouthpiece, and in due time your mouth. You're better off not staining your bong in the first place. Water itself will not stain your bong, so fill the chamber only with water, never with soda, juice, tea, coffee, and contrary to the legendary frat house beer bong, never with booze.

Alcohol very effectively captures cannabinoids, which is precisely why alcohol is used for making cannabis tinctures.[3] That is reason enough not to fill your bong with any alcoholic beverage. Further, you need not study etymology to recognize that the word "toxic" forms the root of "intoxicated." Alcohol is the most toxic of all recreational drugs,[4] alarmingly destructive both to the individual and to society. Further, alcohol that is addictive when ingested into the stomach is even more addictive when inhaled into the lungs.[5]

TESTING THE WATERS

If much of this preceding discussion about water pipes has been news to you, then that news has been good. Now for the bad news, intimated by the statement that alcohol captures cannabinoids. The very water that filters out the bad components of smoke that you want to avoid will also filter out the very things that you seek, namely terpenes and cannabinoids. Most research about water pipes had historically been conducted with tobacco, and only a rare few with cannabis. Those early studies with cannabis had asked different questions than have more recent studies, and so those early studies had arrived at different answers.

A widely cited study published in 1993 compiled and reviewed six previous cannabis studies conducted primarily during the 1970s,[6] the primordial years of cannabis research. Two of those earlier studies analyzed the spent water for only the captured THC, not for the full entourage of more than a hundred other cannabinoids and certainly none of the terpenes. Back then, few other cannabinoids or terpenes had even been identified in cannabis. The review study concluded that much tar was captured, but only some THC. Either assured by or oblivious to the study, stoners merrily continued toking away on their bongs.

The most newsworthy water pipe and cannabis study that challenged many popularly held assumptions was published in 1996. Rather than focus on THC alone, it tested the spent waters for the full range of total cannabinoids. It found that water pipes filtered out proportionately more cannabinoids than tar, which were more cannabinoids than were previously studied. It proposed that to compensate, water pipe users would end up smoking more, and therefore inhaling more tars, to reach their desired effect.[7] With smokers right back where they started in regard to total intake of tars and other toxins, the potential benefit reaped from a water pipe was counterproductive and was canceled out.[8] Such a prospect surely proved disappointing to water pipe users who preferred its milder smoke, and who had assumed that smoking with a water pipe also presented fewer health risks than with a hand pipe or a rolled joint.

This quandary about the ratio of captured tar to captured cannabinoids presently lacks any definitive answer, may have no answer lurking on the horizon, and probably never will be answered. The jury is out, probably forever, because there is no jury. That 1996 study was the last of its kind. A harm reduction study published in 2015 cited the 1996 study, but it conducted no further research and so added no more data to the issue.[9] It was noteworthy that the more recent study even discussed water pipes. In spite of the plethora of artistic and costly bongs that continue to decorate the walls and display cases of smoke shops, as a subject of research water pipes now go unobserved by the watchful eye of science.

Research about drugs and drug use expands our collective minds but empties our community wallets. Further exploration of the efficacy of smoking cannabis with water pipes has hit a snag because attention has been redirected to the technological wonder of herbal vaporizers. That shift in research has been seismic. There has been a deluge of studies investigating and confirming the health benefits of vaporizers over smoking. If you were considering purchasing a water pipe, you might want to turn instead to the latest generation of vaporizers. In which case, turn to this book's next chapter.

Alternatively, if you presently use a water pipe and hope to continue using one, you can try to reach your own conclusions. You might already be familiar with the animal experiments in other chapters of this book that you may have conducted (you being the animal). Here's another "animal" experiment you can perform.

1. First, clear your head. If you're a recreational user, don't toke for at least forty-eight hours.
2. Measure two equal quantities of herbal cannabis that experience has taught you will be enough to meet your expectations for a single water pipe session, and designate them dosage A and dosage B.

3. Sit back, relax, and switch on one of your favorite pieces of music. Take your time. This is a test, but not a race.
4. Administer dosage A with your water pipe.
5. Make note of how you feel. If you're a medicinal user, have you relieved your symptoms? If you're a recreational user, are you as high as a kite?
6. Clear your head by waiting forty-eight hours, then administer dosage B, this time with your hand pipe.

To achieve the same relief or same high as with your water pipe, did you need to administer with your hand pipe the full measure of dosage B, or do you have some leftover? Anything remaining was the extra amount of cannabis you needed to squander to compensate for the cannabinoids and terpenes trapped by the water in the water pipe. That is the extra smoke that sullied your lungs.

TB OR NOT TB?

Smoking cannabis with water pipes adds one risk factor that has never been linked to smoking with rolling papers or hand pipes. The incidence of tuberculosis (TB) is rare in North America and Australia among Caucasians but continues to be diagnosed among its new immigrants who emigrated from Asia and Africa. In the countries of the West, when an immigrant household or a foreign-born circle of friends regularly shares a water pipe, a high rate of infection with TB can occur.[10] Among these closely knit cannabis smokers who also smoked tobacco, none smoked tobacco with a water pipe. With a water pipe, they smoked only cannabis.

Neither the tobacco nor the cannabis itself was implicated as the source of transmission. The most frequently cited conduit was smoking with a water pipe. Far less frequent conduits included the social bonding of hotboxing (sharing second-hand cannabis smoke while sitting overcrowded in an intentionally sealed and stuffy car) and the sensual bonding of shotgunning (transferring second-hand cannabis smoke while kissing).[11] In all three conduits, the transmissions originated from one of the smoking partner's baited breaths.

Isolated cases of other respiratory diseases have also been traced to water pipes, even when not shared with friends or lovers. Water provides

the foundation of life and provides an incubator for microscopic pathogens that harm larger life forms. Cannabis smokers suffer a higher incidence of colds and flus than nonsmokers. (See chapter 11.) There's no
telling what proportion of the high incidence of colds and flus is directly
attributed to water pipes.

The health risk in water pipes resides in the moist environment that
nurtures the growth of bacteria. If not emptied, cleaned, and thoroughly
dried after each use, the water-filled chamber in the base of the water
pipe provides a conducive environment for breeding bacteria.

Do the TB bacteria carry from the water into the smoke, or do they
find their way "on their own steam" to the mouthpiece? That answer has
not been clearly articulated by the many medical reports linking tuberculosis to water pipes. While the incidence of documented respiratory
illnesses has been rare so, too, had been the use of bongs compared to
other past and present modes of smoking.

TB or not TB? That is not the question. The question is, water pipe
or no water pipe?

KEEPING IT CLEAN

If your answer is, "Yes, water pipe," then you need to be vigilant to
keep it clear, dry, and clean.

Buy It Clear: Buy and use only a water pipe that is clearly transparent, not even translucent. You need to see just how clean or dirty it is
on its inside walls. Leave the psychedelic-colored bongs to decorate the
smoke shop wall shelves and display cases, not your home.

Store It Dry: Rinse and thoroughly dry the entire assembly after each
use. A more important safeguard than rinsing is drying, otherwise a
moist water pipe can become a breeding ground for mold and bacteria,
including TB.

Keep It Clean: As long as you rinse and dry it after each use, you
can consider delaying its thorough cleaning. Delay to once every other
use? Every five uses? Every ten? There is no user's manual to consult
about this. You decide.

As something that we do routinely and without fanfare, cleaning
usually does not warrant detailed instructions or precautions. With a

water pipe, however, cleanliness is a matter of health and safety, so it demands careful attention.

To thoroughly clean the entire glass pipe, you can choose between isopropyl alcohol (rubbing alcohol) and ethanol (ethyl alcohol). If you drink them, ethanol will get you drunk, while iso alcohol will make you sick. For cleaning purposes, the two solvents are interchangeable. But iso alcohol is safer to handle and to dispose of than is ethanol. So better to use only isopropyl alcohol, sold in pharmacies as a first-aid antiseptic.

For sanitizing purposes, instead of alcohol as a last resort you can use household vinegar or just plain old soap and piping hot water. Keep in mind that alcohol is the gold standard solvent that cleanses more effectively and so assures greater safety, especially if you are sharing your water pipe with others outside your household. As an optional ingredient to serve as an abrasive, some coarse-grain salt can be added to the solvent. Salt does not dissolve in alcohol. Neither the EPA nor the FDA provides any guidelines for exact procedures for cleaning bongs. No surprise there. To the rescue, websites that dispense drug lore abound with DIY remedies. No surprise there either. Here is a compilation:

1. Don exam gloves to protect your hands.
2. Dilute the iso alcohol with water. Unless you haven't cleaned your bong in years, straight out of the bottle is stronger than you need.
3. For smaller pipes, place the pipe and the diluted alcohol into a watertight plastic bag, seal the bag, and shake.
4. For larger freestanding bongs with removable bowls and mouthpieces, remove them, and place and gently shake those inside a bag filled with solvent. For the bodies of the large bongs, cap or seal its openings, pour the solvent into the bong, and shake the bong.
5. Allow the bong and its removable parts to soak for at least ten minutes, the longer the better.
6. Remove the bong or its parts from the alcohol, or drain the alcohol from the bong, or both.
7. Rinse the inside and outside of the bong and its parts under running water.
8. Allow all the components to dry thoroughly. The ultraviolet rays of the sun serve as further sanitizers, so if convenient, dry them outdoors under direct sunlight.

SOMETHING TO PORE OVER

Something that all the drug lore websites neglect to address is how to safely dispose of the spent alcohol. If you are very patient and your quantity is very small, you can place the spent alcohol into a shallow and open container. Your disposal problems will evaporate away, literally. For instance, I measured one-quarter cup (250 ml) each of water and of iso alcohol. I poured the two liquids into two identical shallow dishes, stored them at room temperature, and waited and counted, breathlessly. The alcohol evaporated in four days, the water in seven, so the alcohol evaporated at almost twice the rate as water. If water is the sprite tortoise, then spent alcohol is the crippled hare. That's still a snail's pace compared to the supersonic speed at which we zip through our fleeting lives. Waiting for alcohol to evaporate is like a wintery day's pastime of sitting around watching snow melt.

After evaporation, a thin layer of encrustation will be stuck to the bottom of the alcohol container that only vigorous scrubbing will dislodge to enable washing it down the kitchen sink. That's only a few steps removed and one week delayed from pouring the unevaporated alcohol down the drain directly. From there, your drain might empty into the cesspool in your own backyard. Oh joy! Mine emptied into the municipal sewer system in somebody else's backyard. More joy!

Here is where lawyers counsel publishers to admonish authors to advise readers to dispose of iso alcohol in accordance with your local or state regulations. Consult your water district office about the proper and legal way to dispose of spent alcohol. You will likely learn that small quantities of certain household solvents are considered safe to pour down the sink, and that isopropyl alcohol is one of those safe solvents.

The EPA's impenetrable website provides no protocols for pouring iso alcohol down the drain. In the absence of any EPA guidelines, this adaptation compiled from the instructions on the websites of some state agencies and research laboratories will have to suffice here.

1. Increase ventilation in your bathroom or kitchen by turning on a fan or by opening a window.
2. Run the warm water faucet before you begin to pour the alcohol.
3. Keep the water running while you slowly pour the alcohol down the drain.

4. After pouring, flush the sink with at least twenty times more quantity of water than alcohol.
5. Rinse, dry, and safely dispose of your container or plastic bag that held the spent alcohol.

CLEAN, RINSE, DRY, AND REPEAT

If you share your treasured water pipe with anyone other than your lover, always sanitize the mouthpiece with alcohol wipes before passing the bong to your smoking confidant or confidante. Then wipe off any alcohol from the mouthpiece. Your water pipe experience will not be enhanced by the antiseptic smell of a doctor's office.

If all these precautionary measures for cleaning your water pipe and for disposing of spent alcohol have not altogether discouraged you from enjoying your pipe, then please do *clean*, *rinse*, *dry*, and *repeat* as needed. Keep in mind that if you're a recreational smoker and you find yourself wanting to use your bong before it's completely dry, then you're probably smoking too much.

Chapter Six

Herbal Vaporizers

Don't Go Up in Smoke

Puff for puff, vaping poses fewer risks than smoking. Yet before proceeding further, we must clear away the dense cloud of confusion surrounding vaping. By vaping, we mean vaping of cannabis flowers and leaves in their natural herbal form. After harvest, their only processing is drying and curing. Water is removed, and nothing is added. Though dried, the flowers and leaves still resemble how they looked when they were freshly harvested. Give a glance or take a whiff, and there's no mistaking their true identity—100 percent herbal, 100 percent natural, 100 percent cannabis.

OUT OF THE FIRE AND INTO THE FRYING PAN

In contrast, cannabis waxes and oils are highly processed and adulterated. As derivatives and concentrates, they bear no resemblance whatsoever to their natural predecessors. Judging by their looks, you would never suspect their origins were botanical. When purchasing preloaded wax pens and vape pens, you never see the waxes or oils, just the plastic and metal of the pens. Prohibition has stymied research about their risks for human consumption,[1] but with prohibition ending the research is growing. Their dangers now are known.[2]

The practice of smoking tobacco was first introduced to Europe in 1586. Nearly four centuries of use and abuse would pass before it was recognized as harmful. With smoke signals smoldering during their mere ten years of uncontrolled mass experimentation, the vaping of both tobacco oils and cannabis oils in vape pens or other handheld vaporizers is now apparent. Same as smoke, they, too, damage the delicate linings of the lungs.

By 2020, e-cigarettes had been in use for only fifteen years. Published in 2020, the first long-term study comparing the lung health of large populations of e-cigarette users to cigarette smokers was definitively able to reach the conclusion that e-cigarettes are only slightly less toxic than herbal cigarettes.[3] No comparable study of those who vape cannabis waxes and oils compared to those who smoke cannabis herb has yet been published. If you vape cannabis oil and you are waiting with bated breath for such a study, read on.

THE GIFT OF SOLVENTS JUST KEEPS ON GIVING

Cannabis vaping oils are more widely used than cannabis waxes, also called dabs, so here we will narrow our focus to concentrate just on vaping oils. While oil can be extracted from cannabis under a high-temperature and high-pressure process that employs carbon dioxide, that process is more costly and so that oil is confined largely to the high-end and medical marketplaces. All other vaping oils, especially those on the black market, contain extraction residues. Those oils are extracted by bathing the herb in a solvent. Often it is butane, less often propane, and gaining more use by the industry is ethanol. Also called ethyl alcohol, ethanol is the alcohol component of all alcoholic beverages, so its minute residue in cannabis oil is considered safe. Propane and butane are another matter. After filtering and evaporating the yellow sludge, some propane or butane residues still remain in the concentrated oil.[4] Propane is a fuel for indoor heating. As you will recall from chapter 2, butane is a fuel for cigarette lighters. Both are cheap derivatives of petroleum oil. As solvents, both are inadvertently left in.

Other solvents are intentionally put in. To assure that the oil will volatize inside low-temperature vaping pens, that oil is thinned with yet another solvent, most often propylene glycol (PG), sometimes polyethylene glycol (PEG).[5] Yet again, both are cheap derivatives of petroleum oil. The first group of solvents acts as extraction agents, the second group as emulsifying agents. In relation to cannabis, both groups are foreign agents.

Used to create theatrical fog from fog machines, PG also adds a smokey sheen to vape smoke.[6] Vape users savor that thick cloud as a desirable feature, so vape oil makers pour on the PG. While the U.S. Food and Drug Administration (FDA) classifies PG as safe for dietary intake in extremely limited quantities in food,[7] food is digested in the stomach. What's safe to eat is not safe to smoke because what's safe in your stomach is not necessarily safe in your lungs.

The FDA hardly acknowledges that cannabis even exists, so it sets no limits on the chemicals used to grow it or to process it. In 2019, in a belated response to the use of PG in tobacco vaping products, the FDA added PG to its hit list of respiratory inhalants that are deemed either harmful or potentially harmful.[8] Enough said.

While 100 percent cannabis oils extracted by carbon dioxide or ethanol exist in the marketplace, those are consumed orally or topically. Vaping oils contain added solvents. Inhaling vaped oils, whether cannabis or tobacco, coat the delicate linings of the lungs with condensation of oils and solvents that in turn irritates and inflames the lungs. The effect is cumulative, so disease and death are not instant, same as disease and death are not instant when inhaling asbestos, radon, coal dust, or of course tobacco smoke. Yet it took only ten years of creeping death tolls among youths in their twenties for their diseases to be attributed to one specific solvent used in cannabis vaping oils. All the other solvents in the oils and the oils themselves simply will take longer to show the effects of their damage to the lungs.

Health Tip for the Use of Cannabis Vape Oils: What's safe to eat is not safe to smoke because what's safe in your stomach is not necessarily safe in your lungs. In time, cannabis vape oils might very well be banned from the legal marketplace and relegated to the dustbin of consumer history. Until then, it is prudent to resist the allure of hi-tech vape pens and highly processed and adulterated vape oils.

BACK TO NATURE

Time now to return to good ol' traditional herbaceous bud. Herbal vaporizers and herbal vaporizing are surrounded by some hype, even some smoke and mirrors, except without the smoke. The very name "vaporizer" is a misnomer. So-called vaporizers sold in smoke shops do not create true vapor, but instead produce something more akin to "smolder." After you stamp out a campfire, its dying embers smolder. After you blow out a candle, its unburned wick smolders. After you insufficiently snuff out a cigarette, its butt still smolders. The words "smolder" and "smolderizer" do lack a certain charm.

Those words also lacked marketing appeal, so early do-it-yourself developers appropriated the words "vapor" and "vaporizer." Early manufacturers took that ball and ran with it. Like an occupying army, their advertising campaigns seized those two words that previously were associated with steam vaporizers. The original and true vaporizers are compact humidifying devices that emit water vapor, also known as steam. Being small, they are effective only for an enclosed area, for instance the hospital room of a convalescent ailing from a respiratory illness. The refashioned noun "vapor" has since been shortened into "vape" and turned into a verb, "to vape."

Ditching etymology and medical lexicons, the name "vaporizer" and the action of "vaping" have become the cannabis industry standard. Cannabis vaporizers more accurately volatize the herb, rather than burn it. Such devices very well could have been called "volatizers," much to Webster's and my 10th-grade high school English teacher's satisfaction. In fact, the Volatizer was an early but now defunct brand of vaporizer that had claimed that very name. For us contemporary cannabis consumers, the misnomer "vaporizer" is here to stay.

Smoking and vaping still share much in common. They offer one timely advantage over other oral methods of consumption such as sprays, tinctures, and edibles. Results from smoking and vaping can be felt only a minute or two after inhalation, meaning absorption through the lungs. In contrast, ingestion through the stomach requires from one to two hours to take effect. Just as smoking cannabis bud differs from vaping cannabis concentrates such as waxes and oils, smoking and vaping also differ from each other. Papers and pipes cost less, while herbal vaporizers cost more. Cleaning hand pipes and water pipes can be easy, while taking apart and cleaning some vaporizers can be complicated. Smoking is simple, while vaping can be complex. Smoking is older, vaping is newer.

A SHORT HISTORY OF A SHORT HISTORY

As a new technology that has emerged and evolved during our very own generation, the history of vaporizers is short.

For centuries, the traditional implements for smoking cannabis were the hand-rolled joint, the handheld pipe, and the handblown water pipe. In defiance of twentieth-century drug paraphernalia laws, these could also be used also for tobacco, so they escaped banishment from the marketplace. Legally and widely available, they were widely used. Not until the 1990s did we see the early development of innovative but primitive models of the vaporizer. During the industry's infancy, vaporizers were marketed for use with cannabis, not tobacco, so there was no curtain or camouflage that their manufacture and sale could hide behind. Consequently, in the United States, early manufacturers became casualties of the punitive War on (Some) Drugs. The U.S. Drug Enforcement Agency (DEA) shut them down.

But crime is fluid, like water in a balloon. Put the squeeze on them *here*, and they get pushed *there*. Some American manufacturers packed up, fled the country, and set up shop in Canada. Native Canadian companies sprouted up, too. With America's population eight times larger than Canada's, the customer base remained largely American, lured by ads in the magazine *High Times*. Some companies were reputable while others flaunted their expectations that consumer fraud was hard to prosecute across international borders. The latter sold faulty products with warranties that they never honored. If customers tried phoning them to register a complaint, their phones went unanswered, and their answering machines fell silent. Their message machines were not the only things that got turned off. So did many customers' enthusiasm for vaporizers. Mine is the voice of experience.

That first generation of cannabis vaporizers proved as ineffective as they were primitive and drew justified ridicule from Luddites and traditionalists alike. Some were short stubs of soldering irons affixed with toxic glues to ceramic bases, or they were little more than inverted cigarette lighters from cars that harked from days of yore when cigarette lighters came preinstalled in automobiles. One inglorious model that called itself the Cheap Vaporizer was nothing more than a glorified crackpipe. Sold only to the gullible by mail order, there, too, mine is the voice of experience.

Second generation models paraded more sophistication, sometimes overboard and over the top. Some looked like Rube Goldberg inventions that the cartoonist Mr. Goldberg intended as satirical jokes. Rube Goldberg inventions were ridiculous-looking contraptions that applied complex procedures to perform simple tasks in needlessly complicated ways. Some of those early manufacturers of vaporizers somehow did not get the joke. Theirs were tabletop models that also came with strings attached, namely their power cords, which tethered them to an electrical wall outlet. Their users, too, were up against the wall.

To the annoyance of impatient patients and recalcitrant recreational users, the cannabis herb took several long minutes to begin to volatize. Quite simply, those early vaporizers sucked. To keep them lit, you, too, had to suck. Unless you kept at it while nearly hyperventilating, the herb promptly snuffed out. That turned inhaling into a workout and that workout into work. Some models emitted foul odors, and the medicinal and psychoactive effects proved elusive and disappointing. Their promise for lowered health risk was realized only because they were abandoned in frustration. Their lack of risk directly corresponded with their lack of use. Vaporizer? More like, vanquisher.

Most of us who tried those early models became unreceptive to any future advancements in vaporizers. Yet advance they did, as though behind our backs. And the scientific research about their benefits advanced, too.

THE QUEST FOR SCIENCE

In 1996, the results of the very first study were published.[9] The very concept of a vaporizer was so unique, if not bizarre, that the study investigated it only in comparison with traditional and more widely known joints and water pipes. When comparing the ratio of tar to cannabinoids, the vaporizer was proven to outperform the water pipe. This study effectively issued closure to any further scientific research about water pipes while it sounded the clarion call for initiating further studies about vaporizers.

In 2001, at the dawn of the new millennium, the same pioneering researcher, Dale H. Gieringer, published a study that focused on vaporization.[10] It additionally compared the efficiency of three models with each other. Their vapors were analyzed, and the three devices were evaluated. The first model was homemade and was not commercially available for wider distribution. The second was a commercial model that was deemed unremarkable. The third was a commercial model that proved highly effective—hurrah, hurrah; but its manufacturer had already been shut down by the Feds—boo-hoo, boo-hoo. Though intrigued and encouraged by the results, potential new users of vaporizers were left in a lurch.

In 2004, a team of research scientists led by Dr. Gieringer published their results from examining the vape from a single advanced model of herbal vaporizer.[11] The study found that its vapors consisted mostly of cannabinoids rather than the hundred other toxins otherwise created by smoking. Those toxins included tar, ash, carbon monoxide, toluene, naphthalene, and a host of other scary-sounding multisyllabic chemicals whose names you would never utter from your mouth,[12]—and whose substances you surely would not want to enter it.

Vaporizer technology by that time had made great progress, so the researchers focused on one leading tabletop model that had quickly garnered a devoted following among medical marijuana patients. Named after the geological formation that its shape resembled, the Volcano was patented in Germany in 1999 and was introduced into North America in 2003.[13] The Volcano still looked like a cartoony Rube Goldberg machine, but analysis of the gas components of its vape proved that it delivered the results that had been sought[14] and so had met the researchers' expectations.

More research ensued, but drug prohibition laws in the United States still restricted all testing to inside laboratories where one important ingredient regrettably was missing from the recipe. There were no test subjects in the form of living and breathing human beings.

In 2007, a pilot study was published that was the first to gain approval from the FDA to conduct tests using real live human subjects. The lead researcher, Donald I. Abrams, was an early advocate for treating ailing patients with smoked medical marijuana. The added element of inhaling and exhaling humans was a tremendous step forward for research. One preference for recruitment was that volunteers should be "active cannabis users."[15] Conducted in San Francisco, the researchers could draw upon a large pool of highly qualified applicants. The study tested the efficacy of smoking compared to vaping in providing the human subjects their desired levels of euphoria. Half-lucky and half-brave, the first-time vaping test subjects were all able to get equally high or find equal relief from vaping as from smoking.

This 2007 study stands out because it analyzed the cannabinoid content in the human subject's plasma, whereas previous studies had analyzed the cannabinoid content in the generated vape cloud. The THC plasma levels from vaping were nearly the same as from smoking; while here with no regrets, one important ingredient largely went missing, namely the gaseous toxic chemicals from smoked cannabis.[16] The majority of those volunteers expressed a preference for vaping over smoking.[17] All of them surely completed the experiment giddy with happiness to have donated their bodies to science.

CHANGE IS IN THE AIR

These studies tested the ability of early models to volatize the cannabinoids without also releasing many of the toxins that were produced during smoking. Other studies comparing vaping to smoking focused on other issues. Two studies reported overall improvements in lung health, one for cannabis smokers who did not also smoke tobacco,[18] the other including cannabis smokers who did.[19] Two more studies reported that from equal doses of cannabis, the blood absorbed more cannabinoids through vaping than through smoking. The first study reported on THC only,[20] the second on cannabinoids generally.[21] All four studies assessed that vaping will spare your lungs.

A Swiss study published in 2016 translated the above results into more practical terms. It evaluated five leading brands of vaporizers. The researchers had picked some winners because, even five years later in a rapidly changing industry, even to this day four of the five models are still being manufactured and marketed.[22] For all five models, less cannabis was needed to achieve the same results as from smoking. The study even suggested, "This is an economic issue in terms of cost-effectiveness,"[23] meaning vaping will save you money.

By 2018, vaping was being more widely adapted, so vaporizer technology advanced full speed ahead. Two significant innovations included battery-powered operation and adjustable temperature controls. Later models added features such as automatic shutoff when temperature exceeded a predetermined limit or when they had stood idle for too long. Battery power freed tabletop models from the table and enabled portable models to be carried in a pocket or a purse. Vape users could now roam freely in the world. No longer coming with power cords attached, many models still came with hefty price tags attached, and still out of reach to all but the most dedicated of cannabis connoisseurs.

While decriminalization and legalization spread across the globe, the vaporizer industry continues to evolve and expand. The differences in models and in their results can be mind boggling and breathtaking. Cannabis consumers now face an overabundance of choices to dazzle and confound. Brands and models in every imaginable shape, size, weight, name, and price range now crowd the marketplace. The current trend favors smaller sizes and batteries with longer charges. At the same time, in their race to break out from the pack and to lead it, some manufacturers view the smog-filled sky as the limit for frivolous bells and wasteful whistles.

One lusterless example of Silicon Valley folly is Bluetooth connectivity to smartphones through proprietary apps. This enables vaporizers to be adjusted remotely. Remotely? Letting your right hand know what your left hand is doing hardly qualifies as remote. Only the iPhone generation, whose cellphones never leave their one hand, could possibly benefit from tapping out commands to their vaporizers sitting in the palm of their other hand. Call me a grumpy old man if you wish, but my rapt reveries while vaping or smoking cannabis are too dear to me to allow myself to be interrupted by the ring or buzz of a cellphone. The ritual of partaking of cannabis should be leisurely and undisturbed. While vaporizers are complex machines, their operation should be simple. Especially when you're stoned.

KICKING THE TIRES AND LOOKING UNDER THE HOOD

Let's take a look at the mechanics of vaporizers. They function by three modes of heating: conduction singly, convection singly, and both together.

Conduction employs a hot plate that contacts and directly heats the herb. The herb closest to the heating element gets charred, while the herb farthest gets heated unevenly. Conduction devices continue functioning whether you inhale or not. Due to these two factors, they can be wasteful of herb.

Convection relies on hot air that flows more evenly throughout the herb. Heat is fanned by the suction of your inhaling. Stop inhaling, and the air flow stops. Convection devices then stop heating the herb. Due to their automatic shutoff, they can help you to be frugal in your use of herb.

Some nonpartisan vape machines combine the conduction and convection methods of heating into one device. All three modes garner their fair share of fans and critics. If you fly solo, you might find convection models annoying when they shut off on you. If you belong to the school of thought that convenience overrides frugality, conduction models might better suit your needs.

The efficiency of all the different types of vaporizers varies widely. Some experienced vapers suggest that even the cloud of vape tastes and smells differently from different models, though that is more likely attributed to their differing temperatures. Across all models, the odor of vape differs from and is fainter than smoke. Likewise, the malodor of vape in your room and on your hair and clothes is only faintly perceptible. Quite simply, vape is cleaner than smoke.

If you're in the market for a model most likely to deliver the cleanest vape in town, merely kicking the tires won't get you very far. Before buying, it behooves you to take one for a spin. For that, cannabis lounges formerly loaned inhouse vaporizers to club members, but in our post-pandemic society their house models have mostly been shelved. Alas, my pre-pandemic experiences at a cannabis club for patients holding "weed cards" proved only that their clogged vaporizers all needed cleaning. My failed test drives never made it out of the showroom.

Closer to home, it helps to have lots of friends who own vape devices that you can sample. During such opportunities, BYOB: Bring Your Own Bud. That way your stash is the constant, so only the vaporizer is your variable. And that way you'll keep your friends. If lacking friends who can share or recommend vaporizers, you can turn elsewhere for advice. Staff members at your local neighborhood dispensary or smoke shop can offer invaluable input, but they tend to stock only a few of the very many models available. For a more comprehensive selection, enter the labyrinth of the internet.

THE VAPING PARLORS OF THE INTERNET

Online smoke shops generally offer brands of vape machines in greater numbers and in a far broader spectrum than any brick-and-mortar store. Remarkably, certain mail order vendors of vaporizers post buying guides or video reviews that are both objective and informative. In contrast, steer clear of blog and video reviews by part-time bloggers and full-time stoners who drop the word "like" in between every fourth or fifth spoken word and who insert empty idioms amid every fourth or fifth spoken line. Those reviews can be more painful to hear than informative to heed. You know, like, you know what I'm saying?

Websites devoted to cannabis that are dependable and accurate founts of information rely on advertisers as their main source of revenue. In their product reviews, their coverage might be skewed to review only their advertisers' products and to ignore the myriad others. Rather than pan an advertiser's product with a disparaging review, they simply don't review it. Reviews of the advertisers' vaporizers that they do evaluate and praise can verge on looking like infomercials. We all know to be skeptical of a publication's review of its advertiser's product, be it of a meal in a restaurant, a digital camera, a bar of soap, or a lump of coal.

The trustworthy magazine *Consumer Reports* has never tested nor rated any of the many models of vaporizers nor is it likely to do so anytime soon. Until it does, that 2016 Swiss study conducted on five popular name-brand vaporizers will have to suffice.[24] Its analysis of the deliveries of THC and CBD was the closest to a verified purchaser rating on vaporizers that has yet emerged from the research community. Four of the five models passed their inspection and scored high in their rankings. Fortunately for us, the one flunk-out has disappeared from the marketplace.

Commendations of four models should not cast disparagement upon the many dozens of competitive models that were excluded from that one study. A more comprehensive survey has yet to be compiled. Maybe someday I will post my own recommendations, once I have sampled every vaporizer on the market. And that will be never.

BUYER'S GUIDE TO EXPLORING
THE EDGES OF THE UNIVERSE

Meanwhile, look for several features to guide your decision regarding which vape machine to buy—and maybe to love.

Look for intuitive operation. Especially when you're relaxing with your vaporizer in hand and are comfortably ensconced on your couch, you don't want to go thumbing through its user's manual to find out how to shut off the dang thing.

Look for quick start-up times. The seconds can pass like minutes and the minutes can seem like hours when you're waiting for your vaporizer to warm up and kick into gear.

Look on portable models for long battery life and short recharging time. While recharging, when your battery must stop to take time out, so must you. Some models with dead batteries that you can't replace on your own require shipment to the manufacturer. That's long downtime. Other models require replacement of the entire unit. That's a downer.

Look for ease in loading the raw herb and in unloading the spent herb. You'll never cry over spilled herb if you never spill it. Likewise, the vaporizer is less likely to get clogged with herb if you never spill it.

Look for coolness. For handheld models, it's nice when they look cool. What matters more is that they feel cool, namely cool to the touch, not like you're holding a hot potato. Also, for handheld models, don't just look but feel for ergonomics. If a potato fits more comfortably in your hand than does the vaporizer, stick with the potato.

Look for ease of cleaning. The fewer components that need to be cleaned, the cleaner you'll keep them. Glass is more efficiently cleaned than are metals or plastics, so the more glassware, the cleaner.

Look for control, meaning temperature control. In the "old" days, vaporizers came with only one temperature setting, and you had no way of knowing what exactly it was. Nowadays, many models can be adjusted to several temperature presets. Adjustable control of four or five temperatures is four or five times better than just one. Even better, many models offer variable temperature control.

"Variable temperature control" may sound ominous, but it simply enables you to regulate your vaporizer in increments of single degrees in the same way that you rely upon a thermostat to regulate the heating or air conditioning in your home. Just as different models of vaporizers deliver different results, so does the same model at different temperatures. Not just for control freaks but also for health freaks, temperature control opens up a whole new world of possibilities.

THE HOT-BUTTON ISSUE OF
FAHRENHEIT VERSUS CELSIUS

Vaporizers with adjustable temperature controls that feature digital displays offer Fahrenheit-enfeebled Americans the ability to toggle between degrees Fahrenheit (F) and degrees Celsius (C). Toggling is essential only for Americans who flunked out of metric system class, and that includes most Americans. Maybe someday the retrogressive United States will dump its antiquated imperial system of measurement, which it shares only with the equally metric-challenged nations of Liberia and Myanmar. Maybe some century the United States will join hands with the rest of advanced civilization and will convert to the metric system. Even all of Antarctica measures its subzero temperatures in Celsius. Even all of England, where the imperial system originated, has converted and joined the rest of the world. Until then, wayward American hillbillies must strain to translate into Fahrenheit all the data and documents in which the world scientific community speaks fluently in Celsius.

In support of their conversion, a beginning reference point that Americans may already know is the book and film *Fahrenheit 451.* Paper made from tree pulp burns at 451°F (233°C) and above, hence the title of Ray Bradbury's novel about firefighters in a dystopian future society where all books were banned. Rather than extinguish fires, the firemen of the future ignited them. All books were made of paper, so they burned all books.

SOME LIKE IT HOT

Reader Advisory: If numbers numb you (that's why they're called "numbers") and you don't give a hoot about what the numbing numbers in temperatures all mean, simply skip this section.

Cannabis outright bursts into flames at temperatures of 460°F (238°C) and above. But it volatizes at temperatures between 266° and 446°F (130° and 230°C). Assuming it can even register that high, the absolute upper limit to set for your vaporizer is 446°F (230°C). But by no coincidence, few vape machines can heat that high. At that hot point, you might as well put away your vaporizer and get out your pipe.

Cannabinoids vary while typically volatizing between 311° and 410°F (155° and 210°C). Some sources say that the sweet spot for safe and effective vaporization is between 355° and 366°F (180° and 186°C). Some medicinal users attest that releasing the CBD at 338°F (170°C) provides them the most relief, while some pothead pundits call 392°F (200°C) ideal for maximum release of the THC. But that's near where cannabis perches perilously close to the edge of burning and when harmful hydrocarbons begin to form.

All these volatizing numbers are measures of "boiling points." Boiling points require some explanation because they don't make much sense when applied to solids, so let's start with what does make sense, namely melting points. For example, you know that the melting point of ice into water is 32°F (0°C) and above, and that the melting point of the Wicked Witch of the West is room temperature. As for boiling points, you may know that the boiling point of fresh water is 212°F (100°C). Carrying over the theme of witchcraft, you might envision a witch stirring a cauldron of boiling water with steam vapors rising into the air above it. Boiling points measure the temperatures at which any liquid turns to vapor at normal atmospheric pressure. The boiling point of olive oil, for instance, is exceedingly high at 570°F (300°C). By design, kitchen ovens rarely bake at settings higher than 500°F (260°C). Any higher is only for self-cleaning.

The points at which solids at room temperature turn to liquids extend higher still. Lead reaches its boiling point at 3,182°F (1,750°C). Glass hits its own glass ceiling at 4,046°F (2,230°C). Gold hits the roof at 5,072°F (2,800°C). Apply ample heat, and the solid turns to liquid. Apply still more, and the liquid becomes vapor. How the heck then does cannabis, a solid at room temperature, skip the liquid state and turn to vapor? That's a trick question because it really doesn't. Cannabis in a vaporizer really does not transform into true vapor, but rather into smolder, as explained in the beginning of this chapter.

Naming the boiling points for the vaporization of a solid substance such as cannabis thus can be confusing and is almost a misnomer, akin to the clearly misbegotten misnomer of vaporization itself. As discussed earlier, the more accurate term here for "vaporize" should be "volatize." In reference to cannabis, instead of calling them "boiling points," we would benefit by calling them "vaping points." Unfortunately, it all boils down to sensible linguistics being overruled by the mad scientists. The definition of the peculiar term "boiling point" as applied to cannabinoids and terpenes is widely accepted by the scientific community, so as smokers and vapers we are stuck with it.

BOILERPLATES FOR BOILING POINTS

Different cannabinoids and different terpenes all have different boiling points (vaping points), so with variable temperature control you can target your favored cannabinoids or terpenes. Terpenes are aromatic oils that provide the distinct fragrant odors that distinguish one strain of cannabis from another. Rather than only chase after THC or CBD, cannabis connoisseurs also know to pursue strains of herb with high contents of certain terpenes. For more about terpenes, see chapter 8.

Boiling points vary at different atmospheric pressures. Here are boiling points (vaping points) at normal atmospheric pressure as compiled from one primary source[25] and several other secondary if conflicting sources.

Cannabinoids

The five primary cannabinoids released from Cannabis:

THC, CBG, CBD, CBN, and CBC
220° to 248°F (105° to 120°C) – THC-A and CBG
311° to 315°F (155° to 157°C) – initial release of THC
320° to 356°F (160° to 180°C) – CBD
365°F (185°C) – CBN
392° to 410°F (200° to 210°C) – maximum release of THC
428°F or less (220°C or less) – CBC
428°F (220°C) – THC-V

Terpenes

The five primary terpenes released from Cannabis:
Pinene, Caryophyllene, Myrcene, Limonene, and Linalool

311°F (155°C) – Pinene, an energizing terpene
320°F (160°C) – Caryophyllene, a calming terpene
331° to 334°F (166° to 168°C) – Myrcene, an analgesic terpene
349° to 351°F (176° to 177°C) – Limonene, an uplifting terpene
388°F (198°C) – Linalool, a calming terpene

Combustion of Cannabis

446°F (230°C) – combustion begins
460°F (238°C) and above – cannabis bursts into flames

ON YOUR MARK, GET SET, VAPE!

If you were some miserly old Scrooge bent on squeezing every molecule out of your cannabis, you could simply smoke a pipe or a joint. You would then inhale every cannabinoid, every terpene, and every toxic fume with some ash and tar thrown in. With a vaporizer, however, the goal is to heat your herb up to the point where it volatizes its cannabinoids and terpenes, but before it begins releasing too much of its toxic gases. While this hinges on the hopeful assumption that its temperature readout is accurate, you can dial in your target temperature on a vape machine with variable temp control.

A plausible strategy for testing any new vaporizer, and for that matter any new strain, is to increase the temps incrementally. Alternatively, you can start high and during each successive session dial down. After several sessions, be sure to clean the mouthpiece and stem and any other parts that get soiled. If you're fortunate, these parts will all be glass. For instructions on cleaning glassware, see chapter 5.

The 8-Session Plan, and after each session take notes

1. Start at 300°F (149°C) for a trial run, like a taste test.
2. For every session thereafter, dial up 20°F (11°C) more.
3. After seven sessions, you've hit the outer limits at 440°F (227°C).
4. Now compare your notes.

Or take some shortcuts. Try the three-stage plan. After the third session, clean all the soiled parts.

The 3-Session Plan, and after each session take notes

1. Start at 320°F (160°C) for a mellow sampling and soft landing.
2. Next time, dial up to 365°F (185°C) for a more elevated and energetic high.
3. Finally, hit the heights at 428°F (220°C) for a possible Sleepy Hollow experience of pain relief and maybe the munchies, ending in a somnolent crash landing.
4. If you fall right to sleep, you're excused from any notetaking.

TEMPER, TEMPER, TEMPERATURE

Manufacturers claim, and user testimonies for specific models do confirm, that vaping delivers the cannabinoids much more efficiently than does smoking. With the right model of vaporizer at the right temperature, the cannabis vape might deliver up to twice the cannabinoids as does smoking. That also means almost none of the tar, fewer noxious gases, far less carbon monoxide, and lower percentages of some of the other unwelcome toxins circulating in cannabis smoke. Most unwelcome of all is ash, which causes inflammation of the lungs, and vaporizers deliver virtually no ash.

But what about vape machines whose temperatures cannot be adjusted, whose temperatures remain constant? THC and THC-A are the crucial cannabinoids upon which cannabis' psychoactive effects most depends, but some models' temperatures deliver those in an unusually low proportion. These models instead deliver higher proportions of the available CBD (cannabidiol), the crucial cannabinoid for medicinal effects. These vaporizers whose temperatures remain constant are more suitable for medicinal use, but less appropriate for recreational use—and vice-versa.

A lot depends upon the model of vaporizer you're using. Just as the effects of the same sample of herb when vaped can differ than when smoked, it also can differ from one vaporizer to another, and it can even differ from the same vaporizer adjusted to different temperatures. While many cannabis users still state a clear preference for the effects of smoke compared to vape, regardless of the model used, advocates for vaporizers suggest that such smokers simply had sampled the wrong models.

WEALTH, HEALTH, OR WHY NOT BOTH?

In early studies with human subjects, researchers allowed participants to adjust their dosages on their own. Smoking packs more punch into each toke than does vaping, so you need less time to smoke than to vape. Participants likely stopped vaping within the same time frame that they usually stopped smoking. That may account for why those early studies suggested that smoking got them higher than vaping. In later studies with constant dosing, vaping was shown to be more efficient than smoking in delivering the cannabinoids, because the high heat of smoking destroys some cannabinoids before they reach your mouth. And when smoking joints, up to half of the smoke is lost to side stream.

Newcomers to both smoking and to vaping typically find vaping easier to swallow. Less heat and less irritation cause less choking and gagging. In theory, newbies also need to vape less than to smoke. With more efficient delivery of cannabinoids, both tenderfoot vapers and seasoned stoners need less herb for the same effect, saving you money in the long run. After extended use, you might be compensated for the initial expense of the vaporizer, if your vaporizer lasts that long.

They do malfunction and they do break down, as does any complex machine. The smaller the model, the more fragile are its inner parts, and so the more prone they are for breakdown. Given the expense of their purchases and their finite longevity, it may never be resolved whether any specific model can actually save you money. More importantly, most models do spare your lungs. A vaporizer's main selling point is health, not wealth.

Regardless of its contents, vape is much cooler than smoke, and so vaping is less irritating on your respiratory tract. One study published in 2007 showed that after heavy smokers of joints and pipes switched to vaporizers, their continued vaping reduced their coughing and spitting and generally improved their lung function.[26] Yet comparisons can be unreliable between the general health of vaporizer users and that of smokers. Compare what? Their numbers of coughs per hour? Their episodes of spitting up phlegm per day? Their cases of colds or flu per year, or of bronchitis or pneumonia per decade? The one constant across both groups is their number of deaths per lifetime.

Nowadays, the same cannabis consumer who chooses to vape rather than smoke more likely maintains a healthy lifestyle in other ways, too. She more likely also abstains from tobacco and alcohol, eats a whole foods diet abundant with fresh fruits and raw vegetables, abstains from consuming fried foods and saturated fats, walks or jogs an hour each day in nature or a park, practices yoga or meditation or both, lives in a rural setting where she breathes oxygenated fresh air, and engages in a spiritual or educational practice, even if only by, gasp, reading a book. So who's to say that vaping rather than smoking was the critical factor in her good health, assuming that her good health was even quantifiable?

If some longitudinal and epidemiological clinical trials with long-term follow-ups comparing international populations of hundreds of herbal cannabis vapers with hundreds of cannabis smokers with hundreds of cannabis teetotalers were being conducted today, the results would not be published for several years to come. As of 2015, no such study was being conducted,[27] and if one since 2015 has been underway, it's been a closely guarded secret. So you must evaluate and compare your health yourself. Record all your vital signs and analyze your bloodwork after one year of smoking cannabis without vaping it. Then record and analyze the same after one year of vaping cannabis without smoking it. You just might smoke the truth out of hiding.

Health Tips for Vaping Herbal Cannabis: Vape only the herbal form, never oils or waxes. When it is possible to adjust the temperature on your herbal vaporizer, take the low road. Take small and short puffs— actually sips. Inhale slowly in order avoid coughing, and same as for smoke, do not hold it in. If your friends are clamoring at your doorstep imploring you to share your herbal vaporizer, just be sure to sanitize the mouthpiece.

THE NEW PARAGON OR PASSING FANCY?

Even devices from reputable manufacturers can harbor design flaws that surface only after prolonged use. Once yours breaks down (and break, it will) or once its internal battery dies (and die, it will), you might hesitate to shell out the cash to replace the battery or to buy an entirely new vaporizer. After all, the buzz from vaping is quite different from the high attained from smoking, and you simply might prefer the high achieved from smoking. (I know that I do.)

Vaping herb with an herbal vaporizer is not a total panacea. As its internal parts made of metals and solder heat up, beware of any possible metal oxides you might inhale into your lungs. That's a high risk especially with vape pens, which is yet another reason for abstaining from vape oils. You do not inhale as many of the other nasty fumes as you do from smoking, but when vaping you still inhale some. You still inhale, for instance, nearly all the benzene as you do from smoking. You might even inhale more ammonia from a vaporizer than from smoking a joint.[28] If you inhale too long and too deeply, vaping can still make you choke or cough. If you vape too often, it can still make you wheeze. The vape from some models can still leave your throat feeling scratchy, same as from smoke.

Cannabinoids play a crucial role in the human body, but neither cannabinoids nor terpenes belong on the fragile linings of human lungs. Neither does any intrusive smoke or vape belong in human lungs. Even if our lungs were evolving over several past generations to safely inhale smoke or vape, that adaptation would be too late for you and me. Vape from even the most efficient or most expensive vaporizers still poses some risks.

When purchasing a new herbal vaporizer, many of us are enamored with our new toys. As those toys become old with the passage of time, you may tire of their novelty. Once you have cast them aside or have tucked them away, you might return to "the classics" and savor the simplicity of toking on joints, traditionally used for centuries, or of puffing on pipes, traditionally used for millennia.

Chapter Seven

Seeking Purity
Keeping Your Drugs Off Drugs

As Socrates might have said, the unexamined bud is not worth smoking. So let's examine the bud. During the past years of draconian prohibition, cannabis consumers had scant knowledge of exactly what they were putting into their pipes and smoking. Only closeted home growers and their most trusted confidants knew. The rest of us were kept in the dark. Even the dim flames from our lighters to fire up our pipes shed little light on the subject.

As if tobacco were not already risky enough, cigarette manufacturers stir an array of additives into tobacco's toxic brew. Taking a cue from the tobacco industry, cannabis growers, too, apply an arsenal of chemicals during the cultivation process, both indoor and out. Eating any plant produced with growth hormones and chemical pesticides is worrisome, but a question hangs in the air. Does chemical contamination get transmitted in that plant's smoke? Or does combustion destroy or neutralize those contaminants? Scientific studies have already confirmed that contaminants indeed do get transmitted in tobacco smoke. Researchers are just beginning to confirm the same for cannabis smoke.

Among the first of its kind, a study published in 2013 analyzed the chemical residue not in cannabis itself but in its smoke.[1] It tested specifically for only three pesticides and only one growth hormone. Its findings weren't pretty. It found all four in the smoke. Of the three pesticides, two-thirds lurking in the plant matter was transmitted into the smoke. The researchers concluded that the pesticide and hormone residues in the smoke may pose "a significant toxicological threat."[2]

They advised that the best way to reduce that threat was to make sure that there was not any pesticide in the cannabis in the first place.[3]

WHAT'S IN YOUR WEED?

In decades past, your dealer typically sold you cannabis in flimsy see-through plastic sandwich bags. Full ounces (28 grams) came packaged in bigger and thicker freezer bags. Those bags were the street standards because they enabled buyers to glimpse the proportion of leaves and flowers to stems and seeds.

In the days before advances in cloning techniques of female plants and in the early identification and removal of male plants, the female flowers inevitably were fertilized by the typically domineering males. If there was just one male or hermaphrodite plant in a patch of forty female plants, the overassertive stud joined forces with the wind and flying insects to see to it that most of the females got pollinated and bore seeds. Happy to add weight to the harvest, growers routinely included the male plants and the seeds even though male plants contained little THC and the seeds nearly none. The seeds came either encased within the female buds or, if dislodged, fallen to the bottom of the bag. To fake the weight, sometimes even dark-colored tiny pebbles were hidden inside the bag. Contrary to popular belief, numerous studies have proven that stones do not get you stoned.

The sandwich and freezer bags were just about the only things about the cannabis that were transparent. Your dealer often spun whimsical yarns about its origin and cultivation. He might have pretended it was Acapulco Gold smuggled under the bananas or pretended it was Maui Wowie flown in by a flight attendant in her carry-on luggage or pretended it was Jamaican Dream descended from seeds from the home grow of Bob Marley's personal gardener. And no matter how incredulous the stories, you pretended to believe him.

In reality, neither of you knew if the contraband was indica or sativa or hybrid. You could only guess if its terpenes were rich in pinene or myrcene or limonene. You could only hope that it was high in THC, and you didn't know or care about any of the other alphabet-soup cannabinoids. The only thing you could be sure of was that the cannabis provided you relief or got you high, if even that.

PESTICIDE-FREE OR FREE PESTICIDES?

Sometimes the quality of black-market cannabis failed miserably to provide either relief or a high. While nowadays some patients smoke cannabis to alleviate their migraine headaches, I recall in my distant past a few odd batches gave me headaches. Usually, I bought it from a friend, who bought it from a friend, who bought it from a friend, who bought it from a friend, who bought it from sources unknown. Those layers of friendships buffered me from any beat deals, and the drug deals themselves caused no one any headaches.

During the 1970s, a few times when supplies grew short in summer just before the fall harvest, I navigated the daytime black market of Washington Square Park. Located in Manhattan's Greenwich Village, the park is surrounded by the sprawling campus of New York University, which lacks an unfenced campus green of its own. As a playground for NYU students in search of recreation in drugs, the park is also a magnet for street dealers. Before cellphones, before even beepers, there were street dealers on street corners all over the Village.

In search of adventure to fill the emptiness of my existence, I would stroll along aimlessly in the park until a tall dark stranger whispered to me the magic word, "Bud!" We then sat quietly on a park bench as I discretely rolled a joint from his stash hidden within a folded newspaper placed upon my lap. While I rolled and lit up, the tall dark stranger kept watch. Nearby, street troubadours gathered around the park's central fountain as they beat their bongos and strummed their guitars. Their music commingled in the air with our smoke. Enraptured by both the music and the pot, pot dealer and the pothead briefly transcended social class boundaries as we bonded during the cross-cultural mercantile exchange of my greenbacks for his greens.

On even rarer occasions, with too many cops patrolling the park, my taking a few token tokes was impractical. I could conduct only a cursory olfactory and visual inspection. Even through the plastic bag, the reek of skunk allayed my initial suspicions. Viewed through the transparent bag, the street dealer's pot looked genuine enough. On my mental checklist for authenticity, I filled in the checkbox for all the working parts. The elusive flowers, the overabundant leaves, the useless stems and twigs, and even the loose seeds all were present and accounted for. So we struck a deal. Later, upon returning home with my booty and toking up, I sometimes was stricken with a headache. Something was hidden amid the greenery that I had not bargained for. What?

By the 1980s, I moved to the greener pastures of Providence where I was able to hook up with two local sources of cannabis that was grown organically in soil and under the sun. Grown outdoors, the sunlight was not filtered by glass. To my good fortune, I was able to cut drug dealers out of the deals. My grower and grocer were one. When talking on the phone, our codeword was "kale." My trusted source was a Rhode Island organic farmer whose kale had made him legendary within the local community of kale lovers. If the Ocean State had any mountains, he would be a mountain man. My backup source indeed was a mountain man who farmed in the aptly named Green Mountains of verdant Vermont. Due to their short growing season before it was extended with the widespread adaptation of hoop houses and high tunnels, few family farmers at that time could scratch out a living solely from the sale of their legal organic produce. To supplement their incomes, many moonlighted with sun-grown extra-curricular kale.

Compost-rich organic soil, daylong direct sunlight, and fresh rural air are three natural components that assure the purest cannabis possible. Such celebrated ingredients went woefully missing in the domestic indoor hydroponic grow rooms when the War on (Some) Drugs had tightened America's borders. The marijuana grown in the great outdoors of New England may not have been exceptionally potent, but it was always dependably pure. And given the choice, I preferred purity over potency. Compared to what they were smoking, my friends acclaimed my stash as "health pot." Not coincidentally, my rare Manhattan headaches never again recurred. That was no black magic spell that had been cast upon that black-market cannabis. That was pesticides.

The varying aromas of smoke from different strains are subtle, and smoke from any source tends to numb nasal passages. So after the first toke, don't expect to smell what you're smoking. Instead of your nose, trust your throat and your head. If just a little puff causes you to cough or gives you a headache, don't blame the herb, blame the pesticides. The proof is in the puffing.

When pilots fly aircraft under conditions with such low visibility that they must rely upon their plane's navigational instruments, they are said to be flying blind. When I bought cannabis from downtown Manhattan dealers, I was buying blind. Black market cannabis was nonrefundable, unaccountable, unregulated, untested, chemicalized, and often contaminated. It's a wonder an entire generation survived exploring those poisoned uncharted waters.

Times have changed. Now you can browse the websites of your local pot shop or medical dispensary and can study their online menus. For a more hands-on learning experience, you can walk into the store to pick up the containers and read their labels. Either way, you are provided with some assurance that what you read is what you get. In some shops, you can even open and sniff. Citrusy lemon your favorite fragrance? Take your choice. Indica-dominant hybrid your preference? Here you go. Is Tangerine Dream, rich in limonene, on your shopping list? Yours for the asking. Is a minimum of 30 percent THC high on your wish list? Your wish is your pot shop's command. You name it, you got it.

In other ways, times have not changed. Many unsavory substances in and on the cannabis still don't always appear on any labels. Indeed, the rap sheet could very well serve as an outline for some of this chapter— herbicides, pesticides, insecticides, fungicides, microbes, heavy metals, plant growth regulators, and polycyclic aromatic hydrocarbons. Even when you didn't name it, you still got it.

KILLER WEED

If you are old enough to have remembered the late 1970s, but not yet so old as to have forgotten those years, you will recall the "paraquat pot" scare that struck the cannabis community. At that time, most of the cannabis smoked by Americans was smuggled north from either Colombia or Mexico. Colombian was destined mostly for the East Coast, Mexican primarily to the West Coast. Funded and aided by the U.S. federal government, the Mexican government aerial sprayed clandestine cannabis fields with the deadly herbicide paraquat.

The crops usually were sprayed before the flowers had either blossomed or matured. As American potheads were already accustomed to smoking a whole lot of leaf, the impoverished Mexican farmers marketed that unripe cannabis anyway. Because sunlight activated the toxic effects of the paraquat, the farmers rushed into their fields to harvest their crops before the drug-drenched plants could wither and turn brittle. Unless the leaves had withered, the odorless paraquat was not visibly detectable when sprayed on cannabis. Pot-loving Americans who were smoking contaminated cannabis were getting sick from it. Prompted by outbreaks of "paraquat fever," drug testing was initiated not by the Feds upon the drug users, but by the drug users on the killer weed.[4] Home test kits of questionable value began popping up on the West Coast black market almost alongside the paraquat pot.

In 1978, random lab testing showed that up to one-third of the Mexican crop smuggled into the States was tainted with that very herbicide that had been relegated into Acute Inhalation Toxicity, Category I, the worst level possible. Swallowing less than one teaspoon (5 mL) can be fatal.[5] The American government bureaucrats responsible for the aerial spraying campaign admitted that they knew all along that paraquat caused immediate death if swallowed or inhaled directly, and that paraquat-poisoned pot, if smoked, could cause lung fibrosis, an eventually fatal disease.[6]

The Feds had gone ahead and sponsored Mexico's spraying campaign anyway. The drug crusaders showed callous indifference to the respiratory health of their own citizenry. Back then, smoking pot signaled an act of social protest by rebellious teenagers, defiant hippies, and racial minorities. In the arrogant minds of those privileged white Feds, their victims should have known that they risked poisoning when indulging in an illegal drug.

The paraquat scare led to panic on the streets among American street dealers and their customers. The pictogram for cannabis is its seven-fingered fan leaf, while the pictogram for paraquat is the skull and crossbones. The cannabis community, for the first time, had learned that their drugs could themselves be on drugs. It would not be the last.

HERBICIDES ON YOUR HERB

Paraquat was only the beginning. As an expansion of the U.S.-sponsored chemical War on (Some) Drugs, aerial spraying continued until 2015 on the cannabis, coca, and opium poppy fields in Colombia.[7] The only difference was that paraquat was retired from the arsenal. Fresh reinforcements of glyphosate (brand name, Roundup) were called to the battlefront—same futile war, different deadly weapon. And like paraquat before it, glyphosate taints the soil for years to come.

In 2015, a study was published that found traces of either paraquat or glyphosate in multiple samples of cannabis grown in the Amazonian rainforests.[8] Glyphosate remained in the soil from earlier applications or was dispersed onto cannabis crops by the wind. If not enough to kill a plant, traces may not be enough to kill an animal, not immediately anyway, but it could be enough to sicken animals, including unsuspecting wildlife—and *you*.

Nowadays, hit-and-run renegade farmers in both North and South America protect their clandestine cannabis patches through manual spraying by targeting the undesirable weeds growing among their desired "weed." Like lightning that is said to never strike twice in the same place, bud-tending bandits have no plans of returning next year to the same site. They don't care about contaminating the soil for next year's crops when they have no plans for one. They also toss aside and leave behind their debris and waste, including their sinister cannisters emptied of herbicides and other pesticides.

Trashing of the environment by guerilla gardeners had long been a plague that festered deep inside the American and Canadian wilderness. That plague has begun to be lifted only as cannabis prohibition, too, has been lifted.[9] As it becomes more legal throughout North America, cannabis is no longer the prime target of mass eradication campaigns, so test samples now only rarely show evidence of herbicides. But cannabis continues to be tainted by a vast armament of pesticides.

A PESTILENCE OF PESTICIDES

"Pesticides" is an overarching codeword for a lot of nasty chemicals. While many consumers assign high rankings to recognized brand names, most manufacturers are happy to *not* hear their pesticides' names uttered in public. They are content when their toxic products keep a low profile, including by hiding behind the generic word "pesticides." The popular news media, beholden to advertisers, appears to accommodate the manufacturers. In the news media as in literary thesauri, the word "pesticides" often serves as a synonym for herbicides, algicides, rodenticides, insecticides, nematicides, miticides, fungicides, and germicides. They also spell out subliminal definitions for the word "suicides."

Pesticides thus provide cover for herbicides that stamp out weeds, rodenticides that poison little furry animals, insecticides that swat dead all manner of flying and crawling and burrowing insects, miticides and nematicides that eradicate all the other tiny buggies, fungicides that destroy or prevent fungi and molds, and germicides that wipe out microbes such as bacteria and viruses. As the old adage advises, if your only tool is a hammer, then the whole world looks like a nail. Likewise, if your every spray is a pesticide, then the whole world looks like a pest.

The application of pesticides is limited by state or federal laws as well as by the economic law of diminishing returns. Pesticides are not cheap. At some point, the cost of the pesticides can exceed the cost of the crop loss inflicted by the targeted pests. Unfortunately, cannabis is such a valuable herb that safeguarding it can translate into a heavy toxic load of pesticides. More unfortunately, laws and regulations that limit pesticides on food crops lag behind setting limits to their use on cannabis.

Years ahead of the United States, Canada legalized cannabis nationally in 2018. Only pioneering Uruguay beat out Canada as the trendsetter in legalizing recreational use. Light years ahead of the United States, the Health Canada agency promptly legislated strict limits to the applications of pesticides on cannabis. Controls were subsequently strengthened. As of 2019, testing is mandatory for ninety-six contaminants, pesticides included.[10]

In the United States, federal law prohibits the use of pesticides beyond what is specified on their labels. Yet, no limits are imposed upon cannabis. None. No labels can specify for use on cannabis, so technically any pesticide on cannabis is illegal. That's only a technicality, because no federal agency enforces the ban on any pesticide use on cannabis. Meanwhile a hodgepodge of state laws takes baby steps while playing catchup to each other in the rapidly changing cannabis legislative landscape.[11] Any feeble attempt here to document the contemporary patchwork of seismically shifting state laws and regulations would prove to be embarrassingly obsolete by the time you read it.

Instead of a voluminous overview, here is one brief snapshot only of the years 2017 to 2021 solely in California. The Golden State turned the tide on the War on Drugs when it was the first in the United States to legalize medical marijuana. Cannabis consumers everywhere today owe homage to the referendum voters of California. Their medical marijuana proposal was voted into law on November 6, 1996, a day that now marks our new era of botanical liberation.

By 2017, California and seven other mostly Wild West states had legalized adult recreational use. While most of those states had regulations limiting the use of pesticides on recreational cannabis, California had none.

In 2018, California remedied its lagging behind and leapfrogged beyond all other states (but not beyond Canada). For now, the Golden State upholds the gold standard for regulations with the creation of its Bureau of Cannabis Control[12] and the passing into law its "Medicinal and Adult-Use Cannabis Regulatory and Safety Act" (MAUCRSA).[13] The Bureau of Cannabis Control (BCC) issued guidelines for pesticides that could be doused on other crops but not on cannabis.[14] Of sixty-six commonly used pesticides, twenty-one are banned from use on cannabis, while forty-five are allowed as long as residue levels fall below certain limits.[15]

In 2019, the BCC released the results from its testing of 15,717 marketplace samples of bud.[16] That's a boatload of bud. It reported that one in twelve bud samples failed its broader guidelines. Derivatives such as oils and tinctures failed at an equally alarming rate. Of the flowery flunkies, one-quarter of the failing grades were given for contamination by the very twenty-one pesticides it had banned. By its own accounting, California's oversight had failed miserably.

Pesticide contamination is the cannabis industry's dirty little secret that has never been little[17] and is no longer so secret.[18] Also disturbing is that the legal industry that does uphold high standards of purity comprises only a small segment of the market.[19] Even more cause for concern, recent research has shown that in addition to pesticides getting transmitted in the cannabis smoke, the process of combustion can create some totally new contaminants,[20] some that combine to become more toxic than the one pesticide alone.[21] Expressed in the vernacular, Holy Smokes!

As a nebulous term that encompasses herbicides, insecticides, and fungicides, "pesticides" warrant closer examination of each of its triads. We already have sharpened our focus upon paraquat as an herbicide that targets plants. Next, we will take some snapshots of insecticides.

INSECTICIDES, OUT TO MAKE A KILLING

All insecticides are pesticides, but not all pesticides are insecticides. If this confuses you, it ought to. In a halfhearted nod to show insects their due respect, the toxic sprays we aim at them alone we call "insecticides."

From among the vast taxonomy of insects, only a few compete for our crops, so only a handful of species do we brand as pests. Yet most insecticides kill many non-targeted species, including our friends the pollinators and our allies the insectivores that consume those insects we relegate as undesirable.

Cannabis is a costly crop to lose to insects, so many farmers ensure against damage by applying heavy doses of insecticides. When applied during the plant's growing cycle, it is during both the vegetative stage and the later flowering stage. For smoking or vaping, flowers are the prized part of the cannabis plant. When tested and analyzed, if the flowers show abundant toxic residues, it's frightening to think what amounts had accumulated on the leaves that were not tested.

Insecticidal munitions are applied even to cannabis cultivated in greenhouses, where swarms of herbivorous insects can flourish in the absence of their natural insectivorous predators, especially birds. To control ever ubiquitous spider mites, for instance, some indoor grow labs routinely "air bomb" their entire complex with the insecticide bifenthrin. Even within legal limits set by the Environmental Protection Agency (EPA), the EPA classifies bifenthrin as a possible human carcinogen.[22]

Continuing the focus upon California as we did with more generalized pesticides, one example of random testing for bifenthrin stands out. In 2009, the Los Angeles City Attorney's Office spot checked just three samples of medical marijuana sold in its city dispensaries. The L.A. testing found exceedingly high levels of bifenthrin. One sample measured eighty-five times the legal limit that had been set for produce. In a second sample, 1,600 times the legal limit was found.[23]

In 2016, fully half of all samples from Californian medical dispensaries contained the insecticides abamectin and bifenazate.[24] No surprise there, because those are the two most commonly identified insecticides used on cannabis grown in other states, too. If you don't recognize either abamectin or bifenazate as a household name, there's no surprise there either. The EPA approves them for use only on ornamental plants. Neither is approved for home or commercial use on fruits or vegetables intended for human consumption. They are banned because both are recognized as toxic to mammals, which means harmful to humans.

Both the 2009 and the 2016 tests were performed when only medicinal use was legal in California, thus before its Bureau of Cannabis Control (BCC) was established. If you thought that a medication intended for ill or frail patients would be safe, you'd be wrong.

Even after the BCC began testing for pesticide residues, the problem of insecticide contamination has persisted. During the first year of testing in 2018, an average of 5.6 percent of legal cannabis failed.[25] Testing is costly. One study in 2020 estimated that the total cost for one grower came to a sky-high $791 per pound (454 grams).[26] The study estimated the average cost for most growers was more down to earth at $136 per pound, accounting for 10 percent of the wholesale price of legal cannabis.[27] Market loss due to rejection for failure to pass inspection adds further costs.

Licensed growers, if unscrupulous, may thwart rejection of their crop by simply switching to other equally hazardous insecticides that they expect will not be tested. After all, the BCC gives away its game plan by publishing the list of what it will test for.

Unlicensed growers, scrupulous or not, avoid both testing and taxes. By thus reducing their expenses, they can lower their prices or can increase their profits, and likely both. It's the American way! Even in states such as California where recreational cannabis is legal, guerilla growers tap into the black market through the same underground channels that they may have already tread during prohibition. Even where legal, an untold segment of the clandestine cannabis crop continues to be tainted by all manner of untested and so undetected pesticides. Whenever bootleg bud is sold, buyer beware!

Buying Tip for Cannabis: Know your grower. If you don't know or can't trust your grower, purchase only from legal, vetted, and tested sources.

CAPTAIN NEEM OIL

When smoked, insecticide add-ons are, of course, highly suspected of causing irritation to the throat and lungs, but also of causing nausea, headaches, dizziness, and vomiting. Are organics a safe alternative? Not always. USDA certification for organically grown fruits and vegetables allows for the use of organically based pesticides. Fair enough. When you bring home from the farmers market some cukes or tomatoes, you might not be very effective in washing off the organic pesticides from their surfaces, but at least you can try. You can't even try to wash them off cannabis. When you smoke cannabis tainted with an insecticide, the insecticide can enter your bloodstream more directly than when you eat it. So what might be considered safe to eat and ingest into the digestive tract is not necessarily safe to smoke and inhale into the lungs.

Neem oil is an insecticide widely used in fields and greenhouses to suppress insects, particularly spider mites, to which cannabis is especially vulnerable. The word "neem" resonates with an exotic ring to the ears, sounding like something that Merlin might pull out of his magic hat. Likewise, if not conjuring underwater images of Captain Nemo, "neem oil" evokes something Merlin might rub on his body to make himself invisible. As it turns out, organic farmers apply neem oil to make insects disappear.

Extracted from the seeds of the neem tree, a lilac that grows in India, neem oil is deemed natural and organic by the Organic Materials Review Institute (OMRI) that sets the gold standards for soils, fertilizers, and pesticides. Neem oil contains a toxin called azadirachtin. If ingested directly and, one assumes only accidentally, by mouth, azadirachtin concentrated from neem oil causes severe and constant vomiting in humans.[28]

Urushiol oil, the irritant lurking in poison ivy, is natural and organic, too. No need to touch poison ivy to be poisoned by it. Just briefly inhaling the outdoor smoke from poison ivy during controlled field burnings or out-of-control forest fires causes severe inflammation of the lungs that suffocates people.[29] Yet for smoking cannabis tainted with neem oil, no clinical studies with human trials have determined what possible effects to expect.

DNA VERSUS THC

Patients and pundits within the cannabis community suggest what to expect. They theorize that neem oil is responsible for cannabis hyperemesis syndrome (CHS), a mysterious affliction that has stricken some long-term and heavy cannabis smokers.[30] Symptoms include nausea and abdominal pain, but its signature symptom is vomiting. Ironically, when untainted by neem oil, cannabis is well known as an antiemetic drug.

CHS was first chronicled and studied in 2004.[31] The syndrome spread worldwide and was documented in several more medical reports and studies, culminating in 2012 with a very detailed study of the largest number of cases.[32] None of the studies offered any explanation for the sudden onset of the illness after years of underlying heavy cannabis smoking. And none made any mention of neem oil.

The neem oil theory gained traction around 2015. The notion is that CHS is a reaction to poisoning from neem oil's toxin, azadirachtin, by smoking it. By 2016, the popular news media seized upon the vomiting aspect and spread the story far and wide.

One well-known cannabis researcher and longtime proponent of medical marijuana has disputed the neem oil connection. A veritable member of our home team, neurologist Ethan Russo cautioned against shifting the blame away from cannabis and onto neem oil. Dr. Russo advised that some heavy cannabis smokers have suffered the syndrome where not a trace of neem oil was anywhere to be found. He emphasized that the only sure cure for CHS is to abstain not just from smoking cannabis but from consuming cannabis altogether.[33]

In 2020, to try to root out the cause of the illness, Dr. Russo and his colleagues initiated an international study of cannabis consumers who suffered from it. Enrollees were advised from the start that they were being solicited to provide samples of their DNA. But when eventually faced with the DNA test kit in hand, many balked. Maybe they felt like criminals. Three-quarters dropped out from the study. The remaining study subset of patients and controls was too limited for the researchers to draw any definitive conclusions.[34]

While their research is still inconclusive, the researchers speculated that the disease may have been lurking in the patients' genes and that the consumption of too much cannabis only triggered it. This tentative explanation lacks the sex appeal and sensationalism of the neem oil connection. The news media has not gone abuzz with this story, so in the public's mind neem oil still takes the blame.

Health Tip for Heavy Smokers: Even if clinical studies definitively disprove the neem oil connection, prudence calls for both light and heavy smokers to avoid cannabis sprayed with any insecticide whatsoever, natural or not, organic or not. Indeed, for a host of other reasons, it is prudent to reduce heavy smoking, too.

FUNGICIDES, MY-OH-MY OH MYCLOBUTANIL

Given the choice, which would you prefer to eat? Fungus on your produce or fungicides in your produce? And which would you prefer to smoke? Fungus on your cannabis or fungicides in your cannabis? These questions are largely rhetorical because, unless we grew these ourselves, we are seldom faced with such choices. Rather, the growers usually make these decisions for us. As they often choose the fungicides, all we can choose are our growers.

Using the same playbook for fungicides as we did for pesticides and insecticides, here we'll focus upon California alone. Likewise, from among the two primary fungicides applied worldwide to prevent fungal infections to cannabis, here we'll zero in upon myclobutanil alone.

In 2017, NBC-TV in Los Angeles investigated the cannabis products sold in fifteen medical marijuana dispensaries.[35] The news team sent forty-four random samples to a testing lab. The scorecard for 2017 showed the same dismal results as the 2009 and 2016 random samplings cited earlier in this chapter. The 2017 spot check was one year before California's BCC had placed legal limits on any pesticides. Measured by limits that had been set by California's neighboring states, lab analysis showed that forty-one of the forty-four samples failed their pesticides standards for cannabis.

In twenty-three of those forty-one flunked samples, the fungicide myclobutanil was found, and not just traces, but sometimes in high doses. When heated or burned, myclobutanil was long known to produce toxic fumes, including hydrogen chloride and hydrogen cyanide, which are deadly to inhale.[36] In fact, hydrogen cyanide had been one of the chemicals used in gas chambers to execute death row inmates.[37]

Because myclobutanil's toxicity multiplies when burned, it is totally banned for use on cannabis crops in Canada, in most states that regulate pesticide use on cannabis, and now in California.[38] Yet, in unregulated states, myclobutanil is still routinely applied to cannabis, especially in cold climates where much is grown indoors.[39] Indoors, in the absence of wind that would naturally reduce fungus growth, the use of myclobutanil increases. And in the absence of rainfall that naturally washes away fungicides, the concentration of myclobutanil deepens. After a single application, residue remains in the leaves and flowers for up to three months, which can exceed the life span of the cannabis plant. Let's hope that the life span of the mindful cannabis smoker exceeds that of a cannabis plant.

Health Tip for Avoiding Fungicides: When given the choice in an unregulated marketplace, seek cannabis that was grown outdoors, as that is less likely to have been bombed by fungicides, among them myclobutanil.

MICROBES UNDER THE MICROSCOPE

The same as any other living and growing plant, when alive and flourishing the cannabis plant hosts many viruses, bacteria, protozoa, fungi, yeasts, molds, and mildews—in a word, microorganisms. And in a shorter word, microbes.

In the absence of fungicides and germicides, microbes will be found everywhere, on everything we touch, in everything we eat, in every breath we take, and on every bud we smoke. Humans are not the only usual suspects responsible for adding questionable substances to cannabis. Mother Nature, too, can creep us out when she contributes her fair share of microbes. While most microbes are as oblivious to our existences as we are to theirs, some benefit us, and some cause us harm. The ones that can harm us we brand as "pathogens."

More pathogens lurk outdoors in nature than indoors in the sanitized grow labs and grow rooms where most commercial cannabis is cultivated. While the ultraviolet component of natural sunlight acts as a sanitizer that neutralizes many of those microbes, indoor artificial lighting emits little or no ultraviolet waves. When comparing microbial contamination, it's a tossup as to whether it is safer to grow cannabis indoors or out.

If not the safest, then the most prized varieties according to many cannabis connoisseurs are those grown organically in soil and under the sun. Yet few states allow for legal outdoor cultivation. In most legal states, cannabis must be grown indoors under lock and key. That often means growing hydroponically with lifeless liquid chemicals, so no soil and no organics. One litmus test, so to speak, of organic soil is an abundance of living microorganisms. In the soil, microorganisms are our friends. Above ground, other microorganisms can be our adversaries.

In the United States, states that regulate and test cannabis do not all agree on which microbial contaminants pose health risks. Because testing can be expensive and every test for every single toxin adds to costs, neither do states agree on which toxic microbes are worth testing for.[40] It's hit or miss for safety testing, depending upon where you happen to legally obtain your cannabis. In regard to its inspection for infection, here we'll continue shining a spotlight on California.

In 2019, when its BCC tested a whopping 30,880 number of samples of marketplace cannabis, half of the samples were bud. A total of 360 samples failed because of "microbial impurities."[41] That's one in eighty-six. Be aware that failure was only for cannabis on the regulated marketplace in which the growers knew in advance that their crops were going to be tested. Of the black-market cannabis that was not tested, it's chilling to imagine its incidence for microbial impurities. Time now to stop imagining them and to start examining them. Time now to get out our microscopes and take a closer look at those microbes.

Viruses: While a rare few are harmful to animals, most plant pathogens pose few risks to humans. As yet, there is no documentation of any viruses found on cannabis causing us any harm either by handling or smoking.[42] So viral contaminants of cannabis are in the clear. That leaves us with the bacteria, fungi, molds, and mildews.

Bacteria: Most bacteria in and on cannabis are found amid their roots in the soil. As the roots are the one part of the cannabis plant that we as consumers leave untouched, those bacteria are of little concern to us. But some are found on the flowers of cannabis plants, especially when grown indoors. While the high heat of smoking or vaping kills any *E.coli* and *salmonella* that may be lurking on cannabis,[43] they can pose threats when handled.[44] Best practice dictates that you minimize your handling of raw cannabis so you will not disrupt the delicate resin-rich trichomes, so you now have another reason to keep your paws off your pot. And if you do touch it, as we learned from pandemic safety protocols, it is advisable not to touch your fingers to your mouth.

Fungi: Of the three fungi most frequently found in cannabis grown for medical dispensaries, all three of their toxins can cause lung infections and can be carcinogenic.[45] The most notorious is *aspergillus*. The little aspergillus critters are so resilient that they can endure the low heat of the decarboxylation process of vaping and can even survive the high heat of the combustion process of smoking. Their resistance to heat makes aspergillus especially dangerous to smokers. On one hand, cannabis smoking is considered a high-risk factor for chronic pulmonary aspergillosis, a disease that is difficult to treat and that often proves fatal.[46] On the other hand, the disease only very rarely afflicts cannabis smokers.[47] Phew!

One alarmist medical company that markets its analysis equipment to cannabis testing labs dramatizes aspergillus as the most dangerous of all the microbes.[48] Though aspergillus can indeed infect the lungs through smoking and vaping, not all the states that do regulate medicinal or recreational cannabis consider the rate of risk to be high enough to test for it.[49] As of 2020, only Canada and the six Western states test for aspergillus. To its credit, California is one of them.[50]

Molds and Mildew: Molds and mildews are actually specific types of fungi that warrant special discussion. Molds are the most common type of microbes that grow on cannabis.[51] Regulation and testing do not guarantee the absence of molds, but only permissible limits to their presence. Even with zero tolerance, despite all the testing in the world, once the cannabis passes testing and then departs the test lab, infection can occur. During its transit, its handling, and its packaging, the dried and cured cannabis can still become contaminated by the spores that cause molds and mildews.

Mold and mildew spores are everywhere in the air and can alight on cannabis before or during its packaging. From their spores that are invisible to the naked eye, molds and mildews can colonize on the cannabis inside of the sealed environs of its package, be it a glass jar, a hard plastic vial, or a pliable plastic or mylar bag. Sealing the containers in a vacuum could prevent their growth, but none are sealed in vacuums. Storing the containers under refrigeration can slow their growth, but few if any are refrigerated. Mold and mildew thrive in warmth, especially when above 77°F (25°C). With air locked inside, such uncooled containers become mini humidors in which mold and mildew can proliferate. They can keep on multiplying until the moment you consume it. A childish couplet warns, "Kill it, before it multiples!" We might heed the advice, "Smoke it, before it multiplies!"

Water forms the basis of all life forms. Without water, there is no life. Even arctic ice holds the promise of life. Primitive forms of life though they are, molds and mildews flourish only in the presence of moisture. The potential for spores to grow into molds and mildews is in part dependent upon the level of moisture content remaining in the dried and cured cannabis. Ideally, on its upper limits, it will be moist enough to prevent buds and leaves from burning too quickly and producing a foul-smelling and harsh smoke that can irritate your mouth and throat. And, on its lower limits, it will be dry enough to prevent mold or mildew from colonizing.

Typically, when it reaches the consumer, dried and cured cannabis ranges between 8 percent and 12 percent in water content. Robert Connell Clarke, the Linnaeus of cannabis botany, recommends spot-on 10 percent.[52] Ed Rosenthal, the guru of ganja growing and the author of many books and articles about cannabis cultivation, advises that 12 percent moisture content is tops for smoking a joint that won't snuff out.[53] If you have a hard time keeping your joint or pipe lit because the cannabis is too moist, you should be wary of the high potential for mold or mildew.

Just as food is often recalled from supermarket shelves due to the threat of food-borne illness, cannabis, too, has been recalled from dispensaries and pot shops. At the risk of being blamed for coining a new phrase, this entire chapter could be titled "Cannabis-Borne Illness." Among the roll call for recalls for cannabis, California has had its share, but the recall king for both frequencies and quantities is Colorado. Among all the chemical and natural contaminants that can taint cannabis to call for its recall, mold is number one. Little wonder that the most massive cannabis recall in the United States was for mold in Colorado.[54] It is after the harvesting and drying and curing and testing and packaging and shipping and sitting on store shelves that "Mold Happens."

Health Tip for Smokers of Cannabis Grown without Fungicides: Be on the lookout for mold or mildew. An outright unpleasant odor may signal mold. If it passes your sniff test, next break open a bud. Inspect it under a bright light and peer at it through a magnifying glass or loupe. Mold inside a bud looks fuzzy or slimy. Its color ranges from black to gray to silver to brown to blue. Mildew usually grows on the outside, especially on the leaflike calyxes enveloping the bud. Mildew appears powdery and chalky. Its color begins white or silvery, then later turns to shades of yellow, gray, brown, and black. Though trichomes come in an array of colors, black, gray, and white are not among them.

If you do find some fungus growing on your cannabis, look for a silver lining in that silvery fuzz. Its presence probably indicates that your cannabis harbors no fungicides.

THE LEAD BALLOON OF HEAVY METALS

When heavy metal music emerged during the late 1970s as a loud and booming genre of hard rock, it borrowed its name from the family of elements that weigh a lot due to their dense atomic mass. Back then, hearing the name for that hard rock music brought to mind the periodic table of the elements. Now, unless you're a chemist, the table has been turned. It's usually the heavy metals family of elements that reminds us of that rock music.

The group of elements originally called the heavy metals can become pollutants that accumulate in soil. With rare exceptions such as volcanic activity, the sources of the soil contamination are of human origin. Point the blame to coal and ore mining (the original heavy metals), oil drilling and hydraulic fracturing (fracking), fossil fuel burning (coal and oil, again), farm animal manures (bull shit), sewage spillage (human manure), industrial toxic releases (both accidental and intentional), motor vehicle exhaust (remember the days of leaded gasoline?), chemical fertilizers (pamper the plant, but kill the soil), and good old pesticides (though neither good nor old). Once they settle into the soil, heavy metal pollutants get absorbed by plants rooted in that soil. The heavy metals then bioaccumulate in the plants. If we consume those plants, the heavy metals in turn bioconcentrate inside us. By poisoning the planet, we eventually poison ourselves.

We can absorb heavy metal pollutants from a plant by eating it and, be it tobacco or cannabis, by smoking it. Much research has proven the presence of heavy metals in tobacco smoke.[55] Studies either have taken for granted or are being conducted to confirm the same for cannabis smoke, too.[56] Incredibly, something as dense and heavyweight as a metal can indeed be transported by something as light and ethereal as smoke. The embers at the burning tip of a cigarette can reach 1,652°F

(900°C) or more, which is hot enough to volatize many metals and carry them away in the smoke.[57]

Some plants accumulate heavy metals more readily than do other plants. Called "hyperaccumulators," the cannabis plant is one such hyperaccumulator.[58] When bioconcentrated in the human body, approximately twenty heavy metals prove hazardous to human health. One study analyzed the heavy metal content in the roots, stems, and leaves of cannabis plants grown in four different regions of Pakistan. The study made no mention of flowers, so apparently neglected to differentiate the flowers from the leaves. It found that copper concentrated more in the roots and nickel more in the stems than either in the leaves of the cannabis plant,[59] so those two metals are of less concern to us. Of the terrible twenty, four heavy metals are of special concern to cannabis smokers. These four are cadmium, arsenic, lead, and mercury. The first letters of each just happen to spell the word "calm," which when you think about those metals, you shouldn't be.

Directly through smoking, cadmium poisoning causes gum disease and bone loss in teeth.[60] Cadmium and arsenic regardless of route of ingestion are widely acknowledged to be carcinogenic. Mercury may cause neurological damage leading to muscle tremors. Excessive levels of mercury have been found in cannabis when grown in the volcanic soils of Hawaii.[61] Ironically, because of its mountainy shape, a long-standing brand of herbal vaporizer popular among the medical marijuana community is named the "Volcano."

Lead poisoning may cause dizziness, gastrointestinal distress, and joint and muscle problems and pain. The most notorious case of excessive levels of lead in cannabis occurred in 2007 in Leipzig, Germany.[62] Dozens of cannabis smokers had to be hospitalized for lead poisoning. Dozens more were sickened. Hundreds of other cannabis smokers in the area tested for extremely high levels of lead in their blood. Somewhere along the black-market supply chain, someone had intentionally added lead to the cannabis to add to its weight and thereby increase its market value. Though the study made no speculation about its origin, it is assumed to have been the grower who added it to the soil or directly to the leaves. That aforementioned Pakistani study found that lead in the soil bioconcentrated more in the leaves than in the stems or roots, but that study made no differentiation between the leaves and the flowers.[63]

When a foliar fertilizer is sprayed directly onto the leaves, its heavy metal content can bioconcentrate in both the leaves and the flowers.[64]

Among the states that regulate and test cannabis, only a few impose limits on heavy metal contaminants. To its credit, California is one of those few states. But those limits are only to lead, cadmium, arsenic, and mercury, and limits fall far short of total bans. When regulators do test the harvested cannabis, that is a noble gesture, but a gesture that is too little and too late in the growth cycle. It would be better if regulators were to dig deeper and to also test the soil.

REGULATE YOUR EXPOSURE TO
PLANT GROWTH REGULATORS

Plants on steroids? Not quite, because steroids are synthetic hormones intended for humans. But plant growth regulators (PGR) are hormones intended for plants. Some regulators are stimulators and some are re-tarders. For cannabis, some PGRs stimulate flower growth, while others retard leaf or stem growth as a roundabout means of promoting flower growth. Ultimately, it's all about pumping up flower mass the way that steroids for humans can pump up muscle mass.

Some PGRs are marketed specifically for cannabis and may be in-cluded in hydroponic formulas without being listed as an ingredient. The array of hydroponic formulas that are sold in indoor grow shops is staggering. When marketed separately, PGRs are advertised to promote heavy, rock-hard flowers and dense nuggets, the kind that consumers often seek. When they fatten buds, the buds increase in weight, which increases crop yield and benefits growers. But what benefits growers comes at a risk to smokers. No PGRs are fit for human consumption. Those commonly found in cannabis include carcinogens that have been shown to be harmful to all mammals.[65]

In the United States, in the absence of any broad federal bans and with legal access to PGRs, shady growers for the black market routinely resort to PGRs. For cannabis cultivation, the two most common PGRs used to promote flower growth are daminozide and paclobutrazol.

Daminozide slows the growth of leaves and stems as well as delays the ripening of fruits. It was banned for use on all food crops in the United States in 1989 because of its proven link to causing cancer. Yet, it is still sold because it remains legal for use on non-food crops and ornamental plants.[66] Manufacturers were allowed to continue to market it after they changed its labeling to warn against its use on food plants, which no one would ever dare think of doing. (Wink, wink.)

Paclobutrazol is totally banned in the European Union.[67] It keeps plants short and stocky by inhibiting the lengthening of stems and branches,[68] thus making it ideal for hydroponic indoor growing. While promoting flowering in cannabis, it produces flowers that are deficient in cannabinoids and terpenes.[69]

Tips for Avoiding PGRs: You can be on the lookout for PGR-tainted bud before you even take it home. While tight clusters of the leaflike calyxes that surround the bud are characteristic of cannabis cultivated outdoors, most commercial cannabis is grown indoors.[70] A clear sign of the use of PGR is a small, solid, and tightly packed bud that may seem too heavy for its size. In other words, too good to be true. Visual cues are orange or brown hairs covering the entire outer surface and inner sanctum of the bud,[71] making it look like a hairball that your cat spat out. Deficient in terpenes, when put to a sniff test the bud may emit little or no aroma.[72] Deficient in cannabinoids, if brought home and put it to the toke test, it will barely provide you with any psychoactive effect or medicinal relief, making it all bark and no bite.

AVOID PAH BURNOUT

If you thought that something with "aromatic" in its middle name would be a good thing, you would be mistaken. Polycyclic aromatic hydrocarbons (PAH) are a common environmental toxin. Organic matter is defined as anything that contains some carbon molecules. When organic matter burns, be it wood, coal, oil, or tobacco, that carbon transforms into PAH that then is released and circulates in the smoke. If that smoke is inhaled, PAH can cause respiratory illnesses. As you might expect, PAH indeed are formed in cannabis smoke.[73]

PAH also form in the wood smoke from forest fires.[74] In recent years when the landscape was on fire on the West Coast and entire forests were ablaze, the wildfires emitted vast clouds of smoke that for days on end registered on the Air Quality Index (AQI) as hazardous, the very worst level. Wind then dispersed PAH into the water and onto the soil in the immediate vicinities, including onto the plants growing on outdoor farms of, you guessed it, cannabis.[75] The next spring, PAH also appeared within whatever new plants grew in that soil. In Oregon, Washington, and California, those budding new plants included cannabis.

PAH is pervasive in the environment. It is even on the menu. If you eat food that is fried or smoked or just downright burned, or meat that is grilled or barbecued, you are eating PAH.[76] If you place a lump of meat on your charcoal barbecue and allow its fat to drip onto the coals and that fat to burn and its smoke to coat the meat, then you are helping yourself to generous portions of PAH galore.[77] PAH are especially pervasive in the urban scene. When I spew my auto exhaust into the faces of the drivers behind me, and the drivers ahead of me spew theirs into my face, we are all routinely breathing in PAH.

PAH also coats cannabis when the drying process is hurried by propane heaters.[78] During an extremely frigid wintery night, I have witnessed a large-scale mesclun farm blast portable propane heaters inside its high tunnels where its mesclun salad greens were growing. Fumes filled the indoor air. PAH circulated in that air and onto the salad greens. If cannabis were growing there, then PAH would have settled onto the cannabis, too. Thus PAH can form *on*, *in*, and *from* cannabis: on the plant from smoke and fumes, within the plant when it grows in tainted soil, and released from the plant when you smoke it.

While neither the federal nor state governments have set safe limits for PAH content in food or in cannabis in the United States, the European Union (EU) since 2015 has set limits for it in oil-based food supplements.[79] It's a start, and that start includes cannabis and hemp oils. While testing for PAH in cannabis is neither mandatory nor routine, tests that are being performed in the United States are showing levels in cannabis oils that far exceed the EU guidelines.[80]

Tips for Avoiding PAH: The only practical way to minimize your exposure to PAH in cannabis is to avoid product that was grown or dried indoors near combusted heating or that was grown outdoors near wildfires or in heavily industrialized environments.[81] Even when PAH has not formed in or on cannabis while the plant was growing, they still will form when you smoke its flowers and leaves. The only way you can altogether avoid PAH in cannabis smoke is to not smoke it.

KILL BILL

"Legalization and Regulation" have been the holy mantras of the move-ment for cannabis law reform. Legalization, where it has not already been enacted, and regulation, if it ever is fully enforced, could blaze a path to solving many of the problems of contamination thus far pre-sented in this chapter. Legalization requires legislation or voter referen-dum, while regulation requires government oversight, but in the United States no federal agency even pretends to regulate the widespread use of toxic chemicals on cannabis. The responsibility of lifting cannabis out of its health and safety void has rested upon the states. But in some states, Big Cannabis has followed the playbook scripted by Big To-bacco in thwarting any attempts at regulation.

It is easy to imagine whose campaign coffers Corporate Cannabis has filled when certain recalcitrant legislators cite the protection of free enterprise as their reason for voting against regulatory bills. It's almost a Wild West out there even in the lands of legal cannabis. In defiance of federal law, Colorado and Washington were the first to legalize rec-reational use in the United States. In an effort to protect both consumers and farm workers in Colorado, its governor first issued an executive order and then introduced a bill that would recall and confiscate crops whose pesticide residues exceeded certain modest limits.[82] Recalls would have served as an effective deterrent against the indiscriminate application of pesticides—would have, could have, should have.

Legislators killed the governor's bill under the pretense of protect-ing the property rights of the growers. Newspaper headlines alone tell the story of the ongoing saga. The *Denver Post* reported on the failed legislation under the headline "Colorado Yields to Marijuana Industry Pressure on Pesticides"[83] and the next year, "Colorado Pot Industry Steps Up Pesticide Fight Against Regulators."[84]

The lobbyists for Corporate Cannabis busy themselves in other states on other issues, too. Potential competition from legalized home grows presents an existential threat to Big Cannabis. When New York State was wrangling to legalize recreational cannabis, the mayor of New York City advocated to include home cultivation as part of the plan. Corporate Cannabis promptly stepped in to influence the governor to quash that proposal.[85] More examples of shareholder- and bonus-driven corporate obstruction could be cited, but enough.

Years ago, medical marijuana patients rhapsodized in online forums and political rallies about their cannabis community, while in California patients formed their own gardening co-ops. Now, CEO's tabulate in spreadsheets and annual reports about their cannabis industry. Community has been lost to industry, cooperation lost to corporation. Still, with the proper regulatory oversight, something can be gained, namely purity. But by whose oversight?

ORGANICALLY GROAN

It's coming, if by the time you read this it has not already come. Eventually, the United States will grant full legal status on the federal level to the recreational use of cannabis. Once granted, one sure path to purity resides in regulating and certifying cannabis as organically grown. The trail map to that lofty goal, however, remains blurry and uncertain. For guidance, Americans cannot even look to Canada, a nation far more advanced than the United States in all things cannabis.

In Canada, much cannabis is already being claimed to be grown organically. The question is, by whose standards? The Canadian Food Inspection Agency (CFIA) oversees and certifies organic food products in the same way as does its American counterpart, the USDA. Because cannabis is governed by Canada's Cannabis Act and not its Safe Food for Canadians Act, Health Canada regulates cannabis cultivation. But only CFIA, not Health Canada, provides organic certification. CFIA does not touch cannabis, while Health Canada does not touch organics. So organically grown (OG) cannabis in Canada falls through a large bureaucratic crack and is left wedged somewhere between a no-man's land and a never-never land. As of 2021, three years after cannabis was legalized nationally, no Canadian nationwide agency certifies OG cannabis.[86] Instead, organic growers in Canada contract with an assortment of third-party certifiers, each abiding by its own set of rules.

In the United States, the USDA is charged with limiting the toxic chemicals applied to food plants, but it does not knight with its official seal of approval any cannabis as OG. Hemp seeds intended as food for human consumption can receive USDA organic certification but not hemp flowers destined for smoking. (Smoke shops sell hemp cigarettes, whose CBD-rich smoke is used to treat anxiety and stress.) The USDA also does not grant OG status to the one brand of cigarettes whose tobacco is organic. It labels its tobacco "organic" and can do so because technically any substance that contains carbon molecules is organic matter. But it cannot call its tobacco "organically grown" because, as a drug, tobacco cigarettes are regulated by the FDA.[87] But in the same vein as Health Canada, the FDA does not touch organics, and like the CFIA, the USDA does not touch cannabis.

Among the states, California leads the way here. In 2018, California proposed a law to establish an organic certification program that was comparable to the USDA's. That law was never passed. In 2020, the state forged ahead and proposed to initiate its OCal Program[88] to define and enforce a "comparable-to-organic" statewide standard for cannabis. As of 2021, however, even as only a proposal, it has yet to be finalized. No telling when the finalized proposal will be authorized. Maybe, just maybe, by the time you read this, it will indeed have been enacted. Meanwhile, in California and the other American states where cannabis is fully legal, an assortment of third-party certifiers has stepped in to fill the OG regulatory void. And just like in Canada, each abides by its own set of rules.

The number of third-party certifiers is both encouraging and disheartening. It is encouraging that there are so many and disheartening that their protocols diverge so widely and span across so many states. The one thing they all share in common is their being prohibited from labeling cannabis as OG. They can describe it as organic, but without the "USDA Organic" circular seal of approval they cannot label it OG. The USDA claims sovereignty over the catchphrase "organically grown," and of course the USDA does not touch cannabis.

Among the first to take up the regulatory slack, the Clean Green Certified program was established in the very Western states that were on the forefront of legalizing cannabis. It anoints its program as "the closest to organic that cannabis can get."[89] Another program, Oregon Sungrown Farm Certification,[90] claims that it was the first, though probably only the first in Oregon.

The Cannabis Certification Council (CCC) appears defiant of the USDA's guardianship of that catchphrase "organically grown." CCC does not elevate any cannabis to that high perch of OG, but only the name of its own program, namely the CCC "Organically Grown" Cannabis Certification program.[91] Those quotation marks are the CCC's own and may have been added to cushion its defiance.

Nationwide in both Canada and the United States, the Pure Regenerative Cannabis Movement offers Pure Certification that it boasts "goes beyond"[92] the USDA's. Certified Kind, sounding more down to earth, modestly claims only that its program for cannabis is modeled upon and equivalent to the USDA's organic standards for food.[93] Sun+Earth Certified[94] requires three crucial elements missing from the criteria of all the other programs, namely growing the cannabis outdoors, under the sun, and in soil.

The Cannabis Safety and Quality Certification program[95] is the new kid on the block. As a latecomer, it makes no claims whatsoever for certifying organics, just for purity, the very goal of organics and of this entire discussion.

And the list goes on. Even if cannabis did fall within its scope, the USDA's perplexing standards for certifying what it deems as OG would only open a whole new aluminum can of earthworms because organics is not the final frontier in growing cannabis—your home is.

HOMEGROWN SWEET HOMEGROWN

Where legal and when practical, grow your own. Third-party certification for organically grown cannabis is commendable, but even better is first-party certification of homegrown because then you are the grower, certifier, and end user, all rolled into one. Just as home cooking can be more satisfying, more nourishing, and usually tastes better than any takeout you might take out, so too the cabbage, the carrot, or the cannabis that you grow yourself. What you grow indoors or outdoors just outside your door will surpass any commercial morsel that corporate agriculture can deliver to your doorstep.

While "weed" can flourish like a weed, when left to grow on its own, cannabis becomes woody, leafy, and seedy. Even worse, half of the plants turn out to be male reprobates. Persuading the females alone to blossom with luxurious flowers requires a great deal of care and much human intervention. Growing worthwhile cannabis at home is never easy and not always successful. If you fail, then you will have learned an important lesson to be all the more appreciative of the labors and expertise of the growers upon whom you depend. And what if you succeed?

Ponder a carrot grown under industrialized large-scale monoculture, fertilized with chemicals, sprayed with pesticides, preserved with fungicides, harvested weeks before you eat it, and shipped from a thousand miles away. Now think of a carrot cultivated by your own hands in your own yard or flowerbox, grown if not organically then at minimum grown naturally, and harvested the same day that you eat it. Produce from our own garden will seem to taste better, even if it actually doesn't. As goes homegrown carrots, so goes homegrown cannabis. When homegrown, you can make it as organic as you want it to be.

The photo of me on the back cover or back flap of this book shows me at seventy years old practicing what I'm preaching—sun grown, soil grown, organically grown, and homegrown! The two twin sisters I am cradling in my hands are two months old and just two hours short of harvest. Given a choice between the stick of commercially grown and the carrot of homegrown, I chose to grow carrots.

Cannabis has been the holy herb of Rastas, the holy grail of hippies, and the holy healer of patients. It is now also the font of riches for Corporate Cannabis. Corporation cannabis is grown inside massive warehouses under artificial lighting and with heating or air conditioning that consume endless megawatts of energy. Devoid of natural pollination, plants are feminized mutant clones that are highly susceptible to mold, mildew, spider mites, and other infestations, so they are doused with pesticides that are toxic to consumers and that foul the air and water. In pursuit of low prices, high yields, and sky-high profits, some commercial growers may operate with little regard for the safety of the consumer or for the sanctity of the planet. In contrast, home gardeners carry the torch passed onto them by the indoor guerrilla gardeners of Holland and the Pacific Northwest during the past half century of prohibition. If you are a home gardener, carry that torch with modesty and pass it on with generosity.

Growing your own cannabis teaches patience and gratitude, hence humility. And it assures freshness and wholesomeness, hence health. When a raja who had ruled thousands of Asian Indians aspired to become lord over solely himself, he retired to a small plot of his former estate and ate only those foods grown with his own hands. Monks and nuns will often spend as much time tending their gardens as their souls, and shamans in some cultures do nothing but pray for rain. Not all of us own land for gardens, but most of us have windowsills or even closets where we can grow our own cannabis. "All that is very well," concludes Voltaire's *Candide*. "But let us cultivate our garden."[96]

Buying Guide for Selecting Cannabis: Where legal and when practical, grow your own. Otherwise, know your grower. Choose craft cannabis over corporate cannabis. Whenever possible, seek what's grown locally, grown organically, and grown in soil, preferably outdoors where it can be kissed by sunlight, can be caressed by rainfall, and where it can reach toward the sky as the limit.

Chapter Eight

Preserving Potency

Evading Ephemerality

The very air, light, and warmth that enable living plants to grow and flourish also reduce the potency of that plant after it has been harvested and stored. In dried cannabis, potency quickly deteriorates when it is stored at room temperatures, exposed to light, and in containers permeable by air. Before calling out those damaging elements, let's first take a quick look at the cannabinoids and terpenes by which its strength is measured.

HERBOLOGY 101

After continued use, it is common to build tolerance to a drug, thus requiring more of that drug for it to render its same effect. Tolerance builds with any drug, be it sleeping pills or diet pills, aspirin or heroin, caffeine or cannabis. No talent is needed to develop tolerance to a drug, nor skill to overeat or overdrink or over smoke. Moderation, however, demands discipline and self-control. The less often you imbibe in any drug, the greater it will affect you. The less often you smoke cannabis, the less of it you will need when you do smoke it. That is simple arithmetic.

In a similar fashion, the stronger the cannabis, the less you will need to smoke. Seek pure flower or sift out the low potency stems and leaves. Higher power flower medicates you to the same level, or elevates you to the same peak, but with less huffing and puffing. The less you toke, the less risk to your health. You do not need to master applied mathematics or to study human physiology to figure out that equation. That too is simple arithmetic.

The scale by which we measure the strength of cannabis has changed and expanded. It no longer is simple arithmetic. First identified and isolated during the hippie sixties—CBD in 1963 and THC in 1964[1]—for the next several decades CBD and THC reigned as the primary cannabinoids whose contents were analyzed and tabulated. Most cannabis enthusiasts went chasing after only THC, leaving CBD for the patients. Judging cannabis by its THC content alone compares to rating beer or wine solely by its alcoholic content. Its percentage of THC is merely a measure of quantity, not of quality.

In 2021, at last count 125[2] different cannabinoids have been identified in cannabis, with new ones being discovered every year. Echoing the reassuring words with which Amazon describes an item's dwindling inventory, there will be "more on the way." Cannabinoids are the heavy hitters in the cannabis playing field, with THC and CBD basking in most of the limelight. While their fans may acclaim THC and CBD as their favorite MVPs (Most Valuable Players), without all the other cannabinoids as team players, there would be no ballgame. The entire profile of all the cannabinoids as well as all the terpenes contributes to the euphoria or the analgesia.

Terpenes, also called terpenoids, have become the latest buzzword and the newest benchmark. As though running neck and neck in a race with cannabinoids, over a hundred terpenes have been identified in cannabis. The two even reside together within the same sticky glands of the flower. Unlike cannabinoids that are distinct to cannabis, terpenes lurk within many other plants. Think of the gooey liquid solvent, turpentine, that is distilled from conifers such as pine trees. Both "terpene" and "turpentine" have roots in the Greek word "terebinthine," itself derived from the Latin word "terebinthus."

Terpenes are the aromatic oils that provide different strains of cannabis with their distinctive colors, flavors, and aromas. The bouquets of specific strains are as diverse as those of wines and teas. If the air is redolent with the sweet and skunky smell of cannabis, credit that to its terpene content. In the absence of any strong aroma, break apart a bud and then take a whiff. If still no bouquet, that indicates that the herb may have lacked many aromatic terpenes from the start, or that the herb is so old that the terpenes packed up and left town, or that you have a cold and your olfactory nerves are obstructed. Terpenes had long been theorized to enhance the effects of cannabinoids, but not until 2021 did the first study,[3] albeit one on non-consenting mice, prove it.

Beyond knowing just the proportion of THC to CBD, knowing a strain's terpene profile can provide further insight into its likely effects. Thus sophisticated cannabis connoisseurs look beyond THC and CBD. They are aware that dozens of primary cannabinoids and primary terpenes all contribute to both the medicinal and psychoactive effects, and that they affect each other's effects on us.

This synergy within cannabis, first theorized in 1998, was dubbed the "entourage effect."[4] It has since been validated and its efficacy is now widely accepted within the cannabis research community.[5] The entourage effect provides the educated consumer with a powerful incentive to seek cannabis in its whole and natural herbal form, rather than processed as pharmaceutical isolates and derivatives. The smoking and vaping of whole herbal cannabis remain so popular precisely because whole cannabis equals more than the sum of its parts.

GRACE, BUT NO GRACE PERIOD

Due to oxidation, any dried floral or leafy vegetable, especially those sought for their pungent aromas, lose their potency over time. For this reason, culinary experts recommend consuming dried herbal seasonings within two years of purchase, and of aromatic herbs within one year. Some chefs concerned more about titillating the tongue than nourishing the body even advise discarding any herb or spice that has sat in your kitchen more than one year. The herb or spice was still safe to eat, but it just would not deliver the pungent punch that was their reason for wanting to serve them. As an aromatic herb, cannabis is limited along the same timelines as cilantro and oregano.

When you purchase cannabis from a source that provides contents analysis, the label on the container usually lists the percentage content of the THC (technically the combined content of THC plus THCa), the CBD (again, actually the combined content of the CBD and the CBDa), and with a few of the terpenes thrown in for good measure. If the label states, for instance, twenty-seven percent THC, that number was accurate for when the cannabis was analyzed, not for when you purchase or later consume it.

In contrast, potencies listed on nutritional supplements take into account that over time their strengths diminish. Listings remain accurate until their expiration dates, not just their manufacture dates. When manufacturers follow the letter of the law, the potencies of their products during packaging exceed what they state on their labels.[6] You get more than what you paid for.

The analysis listed on labels for freshly dried and cured herbal cannabis, however, grants no such grace period. What you read on the label is *not* what you get. You get less than what you paid for. From the moment the cannabis was analyzed, its potency begins to deteriorate, especially when exposed to the extreme elements of excessively low or excessively high humidity, high heat, bright light, and open air.

KEEP IT COOL, BABY

Cool temperatures reduce the rate at which cannabinoids and terpenes naturally decompose. No matter how airtight or waterproof or childproof a container might be, the container in itself is not temperature proof. On a hot day, the hot air outside the container also determines the hot air inside it. In addition to reducing potency, heat can further dry out the bud past the point at which the grower dried and cured it. That's because some of the remaining moisture in the cannabis can evaporate into the empty headspace of the container. The further drying produces a harsh and bitter smoke that will further irritate your mouth and throat. Also, the terpenes are thought to evaporate away along with the moisture into the headspace. So fill the container to the brim and keep the container cool.

During the past half century, the scientific community has conducted two-dozen controlled experiments documenting the depletion of THC over time. You might think that the researchers must be having our own interests in mind in their hopes to advance the best practices for proper storage methods to retain potency. You wish. In reality, their data had been rendered to the forensic services of law enforcement for determining the age and origin of seized contraband.

In 1969, an American study[7] was published that was probably the first of its kind. The study showed that whole cannabis samples stored in darkness and in airtight containers at room temperature lost their THC content at the average rate of 3 percent to 5 percent per month. Like reverse savings in a bank account compounded monthly, if that rate remained constant that would correspond to a nearly 31 percent to 46 percent loss after one year.[8] Don't hide your stash under your mattress.

In 2015, an Austrian study[9] was published that compared twenty-nine herbal samples over the course of several hours at four extreme temperatures of 122°F (50°C), 212°F (100°C), and 302°F (150°C). Those sizzlers are more natural for the planets Mercury and Venus or on the bright side of the moon, so the dismal results of nearly total loss of THC are ultimately useless to us. But the researchers did come back down to earth. They froze freshly dried herbal samples for four months at -13°F (-25°C). The results? The THC content remained totally stable. After one year, only a slight loss was detectable.[10] Same as in the American study, the Austrian researchers also studied samples stored for one year in darkness and in airtight containers at room temperature. Their results were "in good accordance"[11] with the American study that indicated a 3 percent to 5 percent loss of THC per month.

FROZEN IN TIME

In 2019, an Italian study[12] published during the waning days of prohibition stands out because it dug deep into time, as well as into the fridge and freezer. For four years, the Italian researchers studied both herbal cannabis and hashish.

We'll skip the hash. Unlike in Europe, Middle Eastern hash has been edged out of the North American marketplace by our own domestic legal cultivation. Further, when hashish is stored in the dark and at room temperature, its THC levels halve within one year, and totally deplete within two years.[13] As hash consists of the resin-rich trichomes removed and isolated from the protective fibrous seal of the whole flowers, during the production of hash the trichomes' direct exposure to air causes oxidation and therefore rapid loss of potency. The more that the plant structure is fractured and disrupted, the more rapid will be the loss of THC.[14]

The Italian researchers secured samples of herbal cannabis from three different seizures by Italian law enforcement just two weeks before the study began. Thus the samples were deemed fresh and in their prime. If straight off the international smugglers' boats or planes, the contraband would have been fresher than had it traveled through the hands of multiple middlemen before reaching the consumer. In the lab, the samples were sealed in airtight containers. Exposure to air was assumed to be detrimental to potency. Though the test results would have been interesting, the researchers did not waste their resources to compare sealed containers with open containers. The sealed containers were maintained under four different controlled environments. The variables were light and temperature.

Exhibits A and B both were stored at room temperature, A exposed to light, and B shielded in darkness. Exhibits C and D both were kept in darkness, C refrigerated at 39°F (4°C), and D frozen at -4°F (-20°C).

If in early fall you've ever stumbled upon some stash that you had forgotten you had left inside the pocket of a jacket that you last wore late spring, you can guess the results. After three months, the study found that in Exhibit A, 13 percent of the THC had degraded, and in Exhibit B, 11 percent. Only a very slight loss of THC was found in refrigerated Exhibit C. Frozen Exhibit D did not lose any at all.[15]

This hallmark study was the first to compare results for refrigerated and frozen, and only the second to lengthen its time span to four years. Its valuable statistics for the remaining four years were unfortunately presented in graphs and charts that were reproduced in a micro-size font. Being difficult to decipher, the following figures are approximations.

After one year, Exhibit A exposed to light lost slightly more than 50 percent of its THC content, and Exhibit B in darkness slightly less than 50 percent. Refrigerated Exhibit C lost 10 percent, while frozen D lost barely 5 percent.[16] After four years, Exhibits A and B lost another 5 percent to 10 percent of their THC. Refrigerated Exhibits C and frozen D had nearly stabilized.[17]

The researchers found that the rate of loss slackens after the first several months and, if refrigerated, begins to stabilize. The high rate of loss during the first few months informs us that the need for temperature control is most urgent soon after purchase. Another important takeaway is that "[f]reezing is the best storage condition to avoid the reduction of the cannabinoids content over time."[18]

Survivalists preparing for the Armageddon when some catastrophe obliterates civilization can be reassured in their paranoia knowing that they can freeze their stash to preserve it, if not for posterity, then for their next several New Year's Eve celebrations. Before stockpiling their cherished cannabis, they first will need to equip their underground bomb shelters with gas-guzzling electrical generators to power their mini-freezers. It might be less costly and more reliable to stockpile a handful of vacuum-sealed seeds and a truckload of fertile soil.

Being stingy with my cannabis, years ago I preserved a prized batch in my freezer at 0°F (-18°C) and memorialized on its label the date I froze it. Rather than intending to conduct any scientific experiment, I was just being miserly. Around once a year for the next six years, I thawed and sampled a small amount in order to luxuriate in my hoarded wealth. For the first four years, every year I felt confident it had retained its same stellar quality. I employed no refractometer or spectrometer, nor gas or liquid chromatogram, nor nuclear magnetic resonance, nor did I send it to any professional laboratory for analysis. To measure any decline in potency, I used my head. I smoked it.

By the fifth year, I thought maybe, just maybe, it had lost some of its umph. The sixth year, after several samplings (all in the name of science) and while in deep thought (deliberated during the ponderous act of smoking), I came to the conclusion that some of its charm indeed had been lost—not much, but something indeed discernible. On that sixth anniversary, I removed the remainder from the freezer. It was not much, so despite my parsimony, the remainder lasted only a few weeks. Twenty years later, I still remember with great fondness that prized strain and still recall with some pride my accidental research in the exploratory science of the preservation of cannabis.

STIRRING THE POT

Before you head to your freezer to store your stash, be aware that freezing can have some negative effects. Freezing can make the moisture inside the flowers seep outward, thus causing the delicate resin-rich trichomes to turn brittle.[19] It is better to leave the trichomes right where they are inside nature's own packaging, protected from oxidation, moisture, and light. Otherwise, once they have turned brittle, if shaken, the pollen-like trichomes can flake off. Do not stir the pot.

And do not shake the container. Do pack the cannabis to the brim so that it does not shift or rattle inside the container. If the container is mishandled and some trichomes indeed do flake off, the agitation can cause the trichomes to fall to the bottom of the container or cling to its sides if the container is prone to static. As damage control, you can gather those fallen trichomes to smoke separately or to simply sprinkle them onto the cannabis in your pipe or joint. Those harvested trichomes in street slang are called "kief." In avoidance of street slang, some medical dispensaries generically call it simply "concentrate." For folks who intentionally produce their own kief by straining cannabis through a sieve, freezing the remaining fibrous cannabis then has few negative consequences.

If storage in your fridge or freezer is impractical, store your stash in the coldest area of your home, for instance in an uninsulated cellar. Just be sure that during the coldest winter nights the area is not exposed to nighttime temperature fluctuations of freezing and thawing and refreezing and rethawing. Likewise, avoid removing your frozen herb from the freezer, thawing it, and then refreezing it. A second cycle can cause your bud to crumble to pieces. The same thing happens to baked food such as bread and cookies that are refrozen and rethawed. That's the way the cookie crumbles. Look at the effect of seesawing freezing and thawing on asphalt roads when water and ice are added to the mix. Pot holes! In this context, "pot holes" are quite the opposite of "whole pot."

Replace the container back into the freezer as quickly as possible. Otherwise, condensation can gather on the outside of the container, which is just an inconvenience. Open and close the container's cap or lid quickly, too. If condensation were to form inside the container, that is not merely an inconvenience. Any condensing moisture poses a threat to the preservation of the cannabis.

One more advisory. Fridges and freezers sometimes are searched by burglars looking to steal sirloin steaks or other luxury items of food porn. I was the victim of such a burglary—ten-packs of professional photographic slide film that required storage under refrigeration. Being obsessive, I had preserved mine in the freezer. So you might want to be imaginative by camouflaging the outside packaging of your stash. Can you keep a secret? I should not be telling you this, which means I am going to go ahead and tell you this. I presently conceal my frozen stash in boxes that originally packaged vegan burgers, something any ignoble burglar would surely disdain and thumb his crooked nose at.

Storage Tip for Temperature Control: For short-term storage, place cannabis in the fridge. For storage longer than three months, place it in the freezer. And because refrigerators create humid environments, first place the cannabis in airtight containers.

LIGHT-STRUCK

Light is the power source for all living plants that harness that energy with their chlorophyll. Cannabis grows in the light, but once cannabis is harvested light turns into its destroyer. Light, especially sunlight, fades colors, even the colors in the dense enamel paint on cars. The lettering on reflective highway signage made of sheet aluminum, even on those signs that face away from the sun, fades so steadily that the signs must routinely be replaced. Sunlight shreds plastic. Never mind the havoc that sunlight can wreck upon human skin.

Exposure to the ultraviolet (UV) rays of light turns beer sour. To prevent that photochemical reaction, breweries either coat clear bottles with UV protective film or they put sunglasses on their brew by bottling it in brown bottles. The brewing industry's nickname for beer gone bad is "light-struck."[20] Similarly, prescription drugs are packed in amber-colored vials to protect the drugs from the damaging effects of light, which reduces their potency.

Light, especially sunlight, will also degrade the potency of any dried herb. Stores sell culinary herbs and spices packaged in clear plastic containers or clear glass jars to lure customers to the beauty of the contents and thereby to make a sale. The last place where the unsuspecting cook should store that jar of dried rosemary or thyme is in the traditional spice rack mounted on the wall above the stove. There, both the light and the stove's heat will assure a hasty demise of the pungent aroma and taste of that jar's contents.

In the past, pundits and experts have debated which was more damaging to dried cannabis: is it light or air or heat? Does it really matter which is worst? All three are detrimental. Rather than try to settle the debate and to answer the question yourself, protect your stash from all three. If you store it in a fridge or freezer, when its door is shut closed, its interior indeed falls dark. The 2019 study, and every previous study it cited, all showed that light degrades the THC.[21] If you do store your cannabis in a room at room temperature, protect it from light. Its container should be opaque or at the very least tinted very dark brown, same as beer bottles.

Even if stored in an open container exposed to air, your cannabis will be better preserved if at least kept out of sight and therefore out of the light. Transparent sandwich and freezer bags are convenient for short-term sales, but they are unsuitable for long-term storage. They are neither airtight nor watertight, they do not protect their contents from getting bruised or crushed, their static charge causes any loosened fine-particle terpenes to cling to their inner walls, and they do not block out light. Even translucent, amber-colored prescription drug vials, while not opaque, more effectively block out light.

Storage Tip for Light Control: Seek the light, but do not store dried cannabis in it. To preserve cannabis, seek the darkness.

GONE WITH THE WIND

Air in general is not the main culprit responsible for decomposition, rather it is primarily the oxygen in air. Oxygen rusts metals, fans flames, ages living cells, and spoils foods. During the chemical process of oxidation, oxygen reduces the potency of any dried herb. The more there is air, and the longer the exposure to that air, the more there is oxidation. As exposure to air has long been assumed to reduce potency in any dried herb, none of the researchers in the aforementioned studies wasted their time or resources to compare oxidation results from sealed containers with results from opened containers. You would be an exceptionally thorough researcher if you found even one study that had made the comparison. In fact, the six-thousand-page tome and scientific manual for food prep makes the same assumption and has only this to say: "Dried herbs are packaged for the retail trade . . . in airtight, opaque containers."[22] No clue there why.

In the kitchen, every time you reseal a bag, or reclose a box flap, or recap a jar, you do so because you recognize that minimizing exposure to air keeps food fresh and tasty. If you insist on conducting your own experiment to prove to yourself that open air turns food stale, leave one slice of freshly baked bread in its bag and another slice out. In one day, that outsider will stiffen with age. To prove to yourself that exposure to air reduces potency and detracts from the taste of dried herbs, don't waste cannabis on your experiment. Instead waste some oregano.

An airtight container that locks air and moisture out also locks air and moisture in. Choose a container that just barely fits the stash, so that the stash fills the container. Filling yours up to the brim with cannabis will minimize the air in the container. Vacuum sealing pumps can extract most of the remaining air from inside but, unless you just happen to have one sitting around, vac pumps are hardly worth their cost or bother. A less expensive alternative might be to flood the container with nitrogen gas to exclude the oxygen before closing the container,[23] except that the steel cannisters of liquid nitrous oxide are neither cheap nor environmentally friendly.

Regardless of what inert gases fill it, the container should be airtight. While no household container is 100 percent airtight, 99.99 percent will need to suffice as tight enough. Flip-top prescription drug vials decidedly are nowhere close. Screw-top vials with cushioned seals on the underside of the lid are only slightly better. In Connecticut, which models its medical marijuana program upon its prescription drug program, all bud is dispensed in those tinted screw-top drug vials. A few are made of polyethylene terephthalate (PET, plastic recycle number 1), but most of polypropylene (PP, plastic recycle number 5). The vials are so small that they can muck up the works of recycling equipment, so local departments of public works implore consumers to keep them out of the recycling stream. The recycle numbers embossed on their undersides are just window dressing. In municipalities that bury their trash in landfills, those drug vials eventually contaminate the soil. Where they burn their garbage in trash-to-energy incinerators, drug vials eventually poison the air.

Some drug vials are shatterproof. With some luck, others might be made with post-consumer recycled plastics. Some meet the U.S. Consumer Product Safety Commission (CPSC) mandate for child-proof packaging. With no luck, these also seem adult proof. And all are wasteful, costly, and ugly.

Still worse for cannabis, plastic drug vials are static-prone and often oversized for their contents, which allows the cannabis to rattle around inside, which in turn causes trichomes to dislodge and cling to the staticky walls. When an oversized drug vial contains capsules or tablets and lots of empty headspace, you can shake its contents all you want, and you won't harm the capsules or tablets inside. Do that just a bit with cannabis inside and you'll dislodge a lot of its precious trichomes, which exposes the trichomes to air and reduces their potency.

In heavily regulated states, clunky and wasteful packaging is mandated by state laws. Growers and sellers might wish to provide environmentally friendly packaging, but their hands are tied, if not handcuffed, by bureaucratic red tape imposed by legislators and state agencies.[24] The smallest quantity legally sold in most states is one-eighth of an ounce (3.5 grams). To package that in a plastic container requires one-half of an ounce (14 grams) of plastic. That's four times the weight of the product. The cannabis industry has a drug vial problem.

In some states, Connecticut, for instance, when patients want to buy an entire ounce (28 grams) from a medical marijuana dispensary, they must purchase eight individual pharmacy vials, each holding one-eighth of an ounce (3.5 grams) of bud. That totals four ounces (113 grams) of nonbiodegradable, nonrecyclable, single-use plastic. Imagine shipping a one-pound (half-kilo) book in a four-pound (two-kilo) carton. No wonder our planet looks like a giant sculpture by Christo wrapped in plastic waste.

Medical marijuana dispensaries in Connecticut by law must maintain two walls of security. An exterior closed door guards the entrance to the waiting room. That's standard for any store anywhere, observant of laws or not. Then a closed door blocks passage from the waiting room to the inner sanctum where purchases are transacted. And another closed door behind the budtenders separates the inner sanctum from the vault where the inventory is stored. Yet, before I have even opened the exterior door leading to the waiting room, I can smell the heavy skunk scent of cannabis seeping out the door and onto the street outside.

Once my purchase is completed, the budtender places my one or two plastic vials of bud inside a discrete white paper bag. Back inside my car, the unmistakable aroma of Eau de Cannabis emanates from the paper bag and hangs in the air. While driving home, I find the smell-o-rama to be very distracting. Upon arriving home, I am lucky that no cop ticketed me for distracted driving. Of all possible choices for hard containers, those sinister canisters are poor ones. If odor is leaking out, then air is seeping in.

CONTAIN YOURSELF

To protect the delicate herb from being bruised or crushed, store cannabis in an airtight hard container, one with a neutral static charge. If stored in a static-free bag, then in turn protect the bag inside a hard container. Tupperware-type plastic food storage containers, though staticky, suffice as that protective outer shell for bags.

The classic static-free hard container is the glass jar. Canning jars, also known as mason jars, fulfill the job description for thick glass jars with secure lids. Jars are only as airtight as their caps. The most airtight canning jars have lids also made of thick glass that are clamped shut. Other canning jars are sold with metal lids, while additional metal or plastic lids can be purchased separately. Metal lids and caps are only as airtight as their gaskets, the pliable inner seal where the cap meets the glass. With age, such gaskets turn brittle, which compromises the seal. That's why you can buy extra metal canning jar lids. Wide-mouthed canning jars are preferable to those with narrow mouths, though narrow-mouthed will do.

For glass jars other than canning jars, metal caps with gaskets are preferable to plastic caps with paper linings. If needed, tighten the seal by adding a layer of wax paper or plastic wrap between the cap and the jar. A jar has no neck, so no bottleneck. To facilitate easy removal of the herb, seek a glass jar with a wide mouth whose cap spans nearly the entire width of the jar. By no small coincidence, this describes the very jars in which reputable vendors package small quantities of herbs and spices. Such jars can be repurposed for cannabis, which after all is just another herb.

Bags that are nearly as airtight as glass and that are durable and compact include mylar pouches and bags, silicone food storage bags, and oven bags. Oven bags, also called roasting bags, are used for reducing the roasting time of meat. Made of heatproof nylon or polyester, they are larger than you really need, but you can trim them down to size with scissors. Try tearing them with your bare fingers. Rather than rip apart, they stretch like putty. Look along one edge and you'll often find imprinted the warning, "Caution. Keep away from small children. The thin film may cling to nose and mouth and prevent breathing." For storage of cannabis, that air seal is a good thing.

Silicone food storage bags are made with food-grade silicone, a silica derivative. While relatively expensive, they are washable and reusable, so multiple reuses can compensate for their high cost. Oven bags are not staticky, while silicone bags are slightly so.

Mylar standup pouches and flat bags are a practical choice for storage. In fact, where legal, pot shops often sell cannabis packaged in mylar pouches or bags. Hemp flowers, too, are often marketed in these. High quality food items are packaged in these plastic film bags, which makes them easily obtainable for repurposing for cannabis. Virginal mylar pouches and bags are sometimes sold empty in smoke shops. Mylar is a polyethylene terephthalate (PET, plastic recycle number 1) resin of the polyester family. Mylar is a brand name trademarked by DuPont in the same way that Kleenex and Band-Aid are brand names for tissues and bandages. Much to those manufacturers' either delight or chagrin, their brand names have been appropriated as generic items.

Though some herb or trichomes can cling to their inner walls, the amount is negligible for mylar that is cloudy or matte. Clear mylar pouches tend to be more staticky. Clear pouches sometimes may not even really be mylar, but merely shaped to imitate mylar. Metalized standup pouches stand out as the deluxe edition, as they are thicker and block out light. One of their sides is made with a core middle layer laminated in between two outer layers of plastic film. The middle layer is aluminum foil that is often blackened on one side. Imitations are made of metalized polyester merely sprayed onto the plastic film. That completes your definitive buyer's guide to mylar pouches and bags.

THE SNIFF TEST PUT TO THE SNIFF TEST

Among the annals of cannabis research, one of the most imaginative experiments was conducted in Colorado, the pioneering state that in 2012 was one of the two to first legalize recreational cannabis. Published in 2020, the study[25] investigated the cue for warrantless searches of cars during traffic stops when police officers detect the odor of herbal cannabis. Real-world traffic stops mingle with competing car odors such as hangtag air fresheners, tobacco smoke reek, body sweat, smelly socks, luxury perfumes, leftover food wrappers, gasoline fumes, and tailpipe exhaust from passing motorists. Amid such odiferous distractions, how accurate can a claim be that a driver did not pass the officer's sniff test? To find out, the researchers put the sniff test to the sniff test.

Two fresh strains of dried bud were each dispensed into five different plastic containers, so ten containers in all. Each container that held cannabis was then paired with an identical container that was totally empty, thus serving as a plasticized placebo. In total, twenty containers. The five different containers included an open bowl, a food storage bag made of high-density polyethylene (HDPE, plastic recycle number 2), a resealable Ziploc food storage bag made of low-density polyethylene (LDPE, plastic recycle number 4), a child-resistant pop-up-top (flip-top) plastic vial made of polypropylene (PP, plastic recycle number 5), and a doubly vacuum-sealed encasing sheet of composite polyethylene and nylon plastic.[26] Notably absent were glass jars, any of the aforementioned three airtight bags, and screw-top plastic drug vials, the kind that stink up my car on my trips home from the local dispensary.

The twenty containers were placed into separate chambers, ostensibly comparable to the driver's side of a car interior. Only one emanating odor from only one container at a time could fill the air, so no distractions. The containers were randomly put to the sniff test by twenty-one seasoned cannabis users over the age of twenty-one who had developed a good nose for cannabis. The test subjects were blindfolded, so it did not matter if they also had developed a good eye for the herb.

The cannabis in the open bowl and inside the LDPE and HDPE food bags was detected with "100% accuracy."[27] Cannabis in the flip-top plastic vial was detected most of the time. Only the doubly vacuum-sealed composite sheets "reduced diffusion of cannabis odor to levels where olfactory detection"[28] was totally eliminated. So the odious other containers failed to contain their odors. After inhaling a deep breath through your nose, slowly exhale through your mouth while reciting this incantation: If odor is leaking out, then air is seeping in.

Storage Tip for Air Defense: The classic among static-free airtight hard containers is the glass jar. Food bags made of mylar or silicone, and oven bags made of heatproof nylon or polyester, are nearly as airtight, but the mylar and silicone may not be totally free of static.

THE DAILY GRIND

Congratulations if you have made some effort to properly store and therefore retain the potency of your cannabis. When it's time to test if your efforts had any effect, sit back and relax and have a smoke. In order to keep it fresh, you've also kept your bud whole—until now.

Whether its destination is into the fold of a sheet of rolling paper, into the bowl of a hand pipe or water pipe, or into the chamber of an herbal vaporizer, the cannabis should be ground in order to assure a consistent and thorough burn with little wasted unburned leftovers. In a pinch, you can crush a bud with your fingers, but then you'll deposit some oily trichomes on your fingertips where you won't be able to smoke them. Better to use an herbal grinder. The trichome oils will coat the grinder's interior once, and hardly any more again. Round disk-like pocket-size herbal grinders made of metal or wood are sold at any smoke shop. As grinding exposes the herb's highly perishable oils to air and therefore oxidation, grind only just before use. While being ground, the herb will release into the air its pungent fragrance. To catch a whiff, you don't need to put your nose to the grinder.

FUTILITY AND EPHEMERALITY

Before medical marijuana was legalized in my latecomer state, for thirty years I honed my survivalist skills by buying an entire year's supply just once a year in late November. That was very soon after my two organic guerilla gardeners had harvested, dried, and cured their clandestine crops. They packaged their full ounces (28 grams) in quart-size (one-liter) Ziploc-type bags. A heavenly fragrance always wafted out of those bags and filled the room.

Prior to crossing state borders with my contraband, I placed their bags into larger oven bags, and then the oven bags into hard plastic food storage containers. No scent was detectable even with my nose pressed against the food containers, so my car remained equally devoid of Eau de Cannabis. After safely arriving home, I then placed the bulk of my booty into the freezer dialed to 0°F (-18°C). I retained a monthly supply of each of the two strains in separate glass jars stored at room temperature and hidden under the cloak of darkness. Around once a month, I replenished that smaller stash. A year later, in October, my dwindling supply always seemed to me just as potent as on the day I first smuggled it home. Apparently, I had mastered the elusive science and fine art of cannabis preservation.

Yet, no matter what precautions we might take to curb erosion by the windswept sands of time, eventually cannabis will age and lose some potency. The fragility of cannabis teaches us lessons in the futility of hoarding and in the ephemerality of all existence.

Storage Tip to Preserve Potency: Loss of potency over time and most especially during the first few months makes it crucial to store cannabis properly. If odor is leaking out, then air is seeping in. Store cannabis in airtight containers and in darkness. Place any large quantity in your fridge or freezer, and for easy access retain only a small amount at room temperature.

Chapter Nine

Water Cure and Green Diet

Every Mouthful Counts

Smoking is only one of three ways of consuming cannabis through the mouth. You can also cook and eat it as you would a food. You can also infuse it into a tincture and then drink it as you would any beverage. After smoking cannabis, you still should consider eating or drinking, just of something other than cannabis. So welcome to the Department of Food and Beverages.

IT'S ALL IN YOUR HEAD

Smoke is both hot and dry, so the very act of smoking, be it of tobacco or of cannabis, parches your mouth and throat. The ignition devices, be they matches or lighters, further dry out your mouth. The smoking of cannabis goes one step further. Cannabis smoke is hot, it's dry, and its THC content inhibits salivation.

Cannabinoid receptors reside exactly where you'd expect to them to be, in your brain. They also are found elsewhere throughout the body, including in the salivary glands of the mouth.[1] THC ingested by any means, be it by smoking or by eating, interacts with the salivary glands and causes them to dry up.[2] You'd think THC would cause more saliva production rather than less, but the science says that it stimulates the glands to shut down.[3] After smoking cannabis, your mouth can remain parched for up to six hours.[4] That's a long time to be left feeling high and dry.

TOOTH OR CONSEQUENCES

More than a mere discomfort, a dry mouth poses a health risk. Saliva dissolves and washes away sugars and bacterial deposits, so any decrease in salivary production can cause or worsen bad breath,[5] tooth decay,[6] and gum disease.[7] Though cannabis smokers risk gum disease more than tooth decay,[8] both can lead to tooth loss. Just take a look at the bleeding gums[9] and missing teeth[10] of crack smokers, notorious for holding their butane lighters to their lips right under their noses while they suck in the fumes. Or rather, don't you dare look at them. The photos of inside their mouths, illustrated in some medical journals, may make you puke, or at least inspire you to throw away your lighter.

Soon after smoking, scrubbing with a toothbrush and rinsing with mouthwash will freshen your stale breath, will remove any deposits of tar or ash that might discolor your teeth, and the brushing will remoisten your gums. While you're at it, you might as well also brush your tongue and the roof of your mouth. Outside of your home, however, thorough brushing is usually not very practical.

Soon after smoking, if your parched mouth and throat are screaming out to be replenished and soothed, restore moisture to your dry mouth by rinsing it with water. Even better, drink the dang stuff. Drink your water straight, pure and undiluted, not as a beverage that happens to contain water. Carbonated sodas or caffeinated drinks, coffee or tea, beer or wine, and hard booze all are beverages that contain water, but they are not water. Just as you should avoid sugar and salt in anything you eat, so you should avoid those two white plagues in anything you drink, and especially in anything you drink soon after smoking.

If you are adequately hydrated, your respiratory tract should remain moist and your excreted mucus thin, despite your smoking. But most people are not fully hydrated. Water is an undervalued nutrient. Fresh water from a mountain spring, a backyard well, or a rainwater barrel is best appreciated unflavored, or rather flavored only naturally, which is to say by nature. Once you develop a taste for pure water, you will appreciate water as the planet Earth's milk, in which case you will be sipping at the breast of Mother Earth. Do become a heavy drinker.

In a pinch, if you can't drink water, resort to a sugar-free chewing gum. Chewing activates your salivary glands. If there's nothing to drink or chew, but only something to eat, as you'd expect chomping on food activates your salivary glands, too. Avoid salty snacks that will only dry out your mouth still more. Best of all, chew on something green and leafy. When you are indoors and at the dinner table, a sprig of parsley serves as more than a garnish to decorate a dinner plate. Its real function is to cleanse the palette after a meal, especially after a dish containing garlic. If you are outdoors, you might consider plucking a leaf from a nearby plant or bush. Whatever the leaf, its chlorophyll is a powerful cleanser and breath freshener. No leafy green nearby? Oh, yes, there is. What do you think you've been smoking? So when sifting through your cannabis, rather than discard that twig or leaf you might earlier have separated from the bud, save it for later to chew on it.

Health Tip to Remedy Dry Mouth: To remoisten your parched mouth and throat after smoking, drink water or chew on a leafy green.

WHEN SMOKE GETS IN YOUR EYES

The longer the stem of your pipe or cigarette holder, the less smoke you will get in your eyes. In addition to the exhaled and side-stream smoke irritating and drying your eyes, the THC itself that you've ingested by smoking can make your eyes feel dry the same as it does your mouth. That's something you might notice only if you wear contact lenses.[11] Some people claim that if they peel onions right after smoking cannabis, their eyes are so dry that they do not form teardrops.[12]

After smoking, if your eyes feel scratchy, drinking water may not immediately remedy that, but merely taking some action can serve as a psychological boost. Prevention is a more effective course of action. Avoid alcoholic or caffeinated beverages for one day prior to smoking, which will also reduce your mouth feeling dry. For that matter, avoid alcohol and caffeine all the time anyway.

Of utmost importance, stay fully hydrated. How to tell if you are? A home urine test of my own creation has proven effective for me. I don't test for drugs, I test for water. I drink one-half of a quart (500 mL) of water. If I feel the urge to empty my bladder within 45 minutes, then I am informed that I am fully hydrated, and so I have passed my piss test.

Comfort Tip to Prevent Scratchy Eyes: To prevent eye irritation, stay fully hydrated before smoking, and drink water after smoking.

SORRY FOR YOUR LOSS

Some tobacco smokers savor cigars as their after-dinner smoke. Beyond drinking water to remedy the immediately parching effects of smoking, consider the "after-smoke dinner" to safeguard against other risks posed by smoking.

Except for the nicotine in tobacco and the cannabinoids in cannabis, the smoke from the two herbs is quite similar. The long-term effects of tobacco smoking on nutrient loss are well documented, but there is little if any research about how smoking cannabis, too, might adversely affect your body's storage and usage of nutrients. As few cannabis smokers imbibe in cannabis as much as cigarette smokers do in tobacco, it is possible that little or no loss of nutrients occurs from smoking cannabis. We just don't know. Until research specific to cannabis is conducted, we could wait to find out. Or rather than wait, we can filter out the information that is specific to nicotine and then deduce the remaining results as relevant to smoking generally.

Certain foods can replenish those nutrients depleted by smoking. In addition to listing below some of the nutrients lost to smoking, some of those foods are paired with them that can help to compensate for your loss.

ACE IT

Collectively, plasma and serum levels of vitamins A, C, and E (ACE) are lower in smokers than in nonsmokers due to the oxidative stress of smoking.[13] The ACE vitamins all are antioxidants that protect organs from damage on the cellular level, and the lungs are our largest inner organs. ACE are the skin vitamins, and the lungs are skin turned outside-in.

Vitamin A plasma levels in smokers are reduced in inverse proportion to their number of daily cigs.[14] The vitamin aids in healing mucous membranes.[15] Count the linings of the mouth, throat, and lungs as mucous membranes. Rich dietary sources include animal livers, the dark green leaves of vegetables, and the orange- and yellow-colored fruits and veggies.[16]

Vitamin C is depleted in smokers twice as quickly as in nonsmokers,[17] resulting in smokers' blood and plasma containing almost half the levels of C compared to nonsmokers.[18] The smoke from a single tobacco cigarette depletes 25mg of C.[19] That's the amount of C in half of a fresh ripe orange. This vitamin is found only in plant foods. Among fruits, citrus and berries excel. Among veggies, any sprout or microgreen provides an abundant source. For leafy greens, the darker the green the better.[20]

Vitamin E levels in smokers show reductions not as much from numbers of daily cigs smoked as from the number of years spent smoking.[21] The vitamin protects organs, for instance the lungs, from damage and heals any damage done.[22] It is concentrated in the oils of animals and plants, so in liver, eggs, nuts, seeds, and the germs of grains.[23] Sunflower seeds excel among seeds, and almonds among nuts.

SHINE A LIGHT ON THE SUNSHINE VITAMIN

Vitamin D is aptly called the "sunshine vitamin." You can make your own vitamin D when tanning or browning your skin under the sun. The D that you produce yourself straight from the sun circulates in your body far longer than when you pop it as a pill.[24]

If you're lazy and prefer to have someone else make it for you, sources from the animal kingdom include fish, the oils derived from animal livers, and irradiated cow milk. Often added as a chemical fortification to prepared plant foods, the vitamin is otherwise absent from the plant kingdom except in wild or specially cultivated mushrooms.[25]

A deficiency is associated with an increased susceptibility to infections in general.[26] Individuals with lower levels of vitamin D are more likely to suffer from bronchitis, flu, and other respiratory infections.[27] To strengthen lung tissue, the go-to minerals that work in conjunction with vitamin D are selenium and zinc.

Selenium levels in smokers are lower than in nonsmokers due to inflammation in the lungs caused by smoke.[28] Simply by stopping smoking, levels return to normal, independent of dietary intake.[29] The very richest source among both flora and fauna is the Brazil nut. It is also found in fish, other sea animals, grains, and beans.[30]

Zinc is a mineral important for the optimal functioning of the immune system. A decrease in serum levels reflects both the duration and the degree of smoking, while plasma levels seem to remain unaffected.[31] The folk remedy of oysters as a sex food to boost virility hinges on its high content of zinc. As the second highest source, pumpkin seeds should get you pumpin'.[32]

EVERY MOUTHFUL COUNTS

As the average cannabis smoker imbibes far less than the average tobacco smoker, the mileage for cannabis smokers will tend toward the very low side of any ranges given for tobacco smokers. So exhale a long sigh of relief.

The nutrients all cited above are not the full roster but are just the highlights. To compensate for what's depleted by smoking, do I need to eat three slender carrots for vitamin A, two small-sized oranges for C, a handful of sunflower seeds for E, a cupful of wild mushrooms for D, one or two kernels of Brazil nuts for selenium, a palmful of pumpkin seeds for zinc, and do I need to eat them all on a daily basis, or can I skip a day? That's a whole lot to keep tabs on. Which would I lose first, my appetite or my count? But wait! There's an easier way.

While few nutritionists agree upon what foods we should eat, most have reached a consensus about what we should *not* eat. To counteract the ill effects of tobacco smoking, one nutritionist and bestselling author unequivocally implores smokers *not* to consume junk foods, processed foods, saturated fats, white flour, sugar, and salt.[33] That's sound advice for smokers and nonsmokers alike.

During just our past two generations, two new food groups have entered into our lives and into our lexicons—junk foods and fast foods. Many of those manufactured substances devoid of any nourishment are only a slurry of sugar, salt, and fat concocted to titillate the tongue. Yet people scarf down that slop anyway, and they suffer for it when they develop degenerative diseases. Just by eliminating white flour and white sugar from your diet, you will avoid most junk foods. Eliminate white salt, and you avoid all the rest. Once you eliminate all the junk from your diet, all you'll have left to eat are the very foods that compensate for the nutrients lost to smoking. And then you won't need to keep track with a food diary or a diet app to make sure you're eating them: simple and easy.

Are degenerative diseases associated with aging linked to diet and lifestyle? You bet your life they are! Like in a courtroom where anything you say can be used against you, in the dining room everything you eat can be used either for or against you. Mounting evidence based on a global study spanning two generations indicates that a diet wholly of whole foods and predominantly of plant foods promotes health more than all the pills in a pharmacy.[34] A whole foods diet not only can prevent obesity, diabetes, and heart disease, it can also reverse them.[35] Food is your best defense, and every mouthful counts.

CHEW ON THIS

We can devote years to researching the crucial life or death matter of nutrition, or we can ignore all friendly advice and eat only whole and natural foods. What defines a natural food? A natural food on your plate looks almost the same as it did on the farm. By such a definition, herbal cannabis is a natural drug. Except for it being dried, cannabis that appears in the bowl of your pipe or the fold of your rolling paper looks almost the same as it did while growing in the greenhouse or in the ground. That earthy sensuality may unwittingly be why you choose to smoke cannabis in its whole and natural herbal form rather than to consume it as a concentrate or derivative, be it as kief or hash, as tincture or spray, as shatter or salve, as edible or medible, as capsule or tablet, and last and worst, as vape oil.

Think back to entourage effect discussed in chapter 8. There are far more cannabinoids and terpenes to be found in whole herbal cannabis than appear listed on the label of any vial. The same reasoning applies to eating whole foods rather than resorting to pills and potions whose contents are restricted to only what is listed. If you cling to your food addictions and are resistant to upgrading your diet, then at least resort to taking nutritional supplements. Swallowing supplements may seem like a shortcut, but actually, it is merely a detour. Food comprises far more than the sum of its few isolated parts. Many other protective but unidentified and unnamed nutrients are found in foods than whatever short list of contents you might read on the printed label of a vial of pills.

Scientists continue to discover more and more nutrients in plant foods that until our generation no one imagined even existed. The newest kids on the chopping block are phytonutrients, found only in plants. "Phyton" means plant, though we might interpret the ancient Greek word to mean "fight on," which is how the word is pronounced. Every plant creates several hundreds of "phyton-nutrients" to defend itself against diseases and environmental stress.[36] Phytonutrients in turn benefit us undeserving animals who eat them.

Many phytonutrients act as antioxidants.[37] Antioxidants protect the lungs against the stressors of radiation, air pollution, and smoke—all smoke, any smoke. The most common specific type of phytonutrient are terpenes. That's right, the terpenes in cannabis flowers are phyto-nutrients. Heat destroys or reduces the bioactivity of antioxidants. By smoking cannabis, we destroy many of its antioxidants. Fortunately, we can eat other plants raw.

Among fruits, berries excel as our richest source of phytonutrients. Among veggies, leafy greens stand out. And cannabis is a vegetable whose leaves gleam with green. Want a nutritional boost? If you grow it yourself or otherwise have access to fresh cannabis leaves, try juicing them. An entire healing therapy has sprouted up around freshly juiced raw cannabis.[38] One doctor has devoted much of his medical practice to supervising patients seeking to drink raw cannabis juice for its therapeutic properties.[39] It is well within the range of possibilities that the next frontier of research into cannabis will show that eating its raw leaves can counteract any harm risked by smoking its flowers. Stay tuned.

Health Tip for Smokers: Smokers and nonsmokers alike should avoid eating junk foods, processed foods, refined grains, saturated fats, salt, and sugar. If you are a smoker who clings to your food addictions, then to compensate for nutrients depleted by smoking at least try to eat generous portions of the foods rich in vitamins A, C, E, and D, and in the minerals selenium and zinc. If resistant to eating those foods, then as a last resort take these six nutrients in their refined or chemicalized forms as nutritional supplements.

Chapter Ten

Don't Worry!

When You Light Up, Lighten Up

In defiance of illustrated books, instructional videos, and new age workshops telling us that during our entire lives we've been doing it all wrong, we are born with an inherent knowledge of how to breathe. Without giving it a thought, an adult female at rest inhales and exhales an average of fourteen to fifteen breaths per minute. A slower breather and maybe also a slower thinker, an adult male averages twelve to fourteen times.[1]

At a gender-neutral respiration rate of fourteen breaths per minute, that's twenty thousand each day and over 7 million per year. By your thirtieth birthday, you will have breathed in and out well over 200 million times. Try *not* breathing for two minutes and, unless you are an experienced free diver or disciplined yogi, you will faint. If deprived of the breath of life for five minutes, you will flat out die.

The breath of life can also kill you. Worldwide, air pollution is responsible for 7 million human deaths each year.[2] And there's no telling how many animal deaths. Perpetually breathing city smog (cough!) every minute (asthma!) of every day (emphysema!) for thirty years (cancer!) will pose a greater danger than toking on cannabis even once a day. Among your daily average of twenty thousand breaths of air, do not worry about those twenty tokes of smoke. Worrying can cause you more harm than smoking.

When smoking and quietly sitting still, savor the moment and relax! Stress can cause you more harm than smoking. If you transform the simple act of smoking into a ritual similar to meditation, chanting, or prayer, you will create a respite of peace and calm amid what might be an otherwise hectic day. While maintaining good health hinges on fresh air, clean water, nourishing food, and regular exercise, above all is peace of mind.

Good health need not mean perfect health. Perfect health is like ghosts. Lots of people talk about ghosts, but no one has ever seen them. If we were perfectly healthy for our entire lives, we would never die. More in sync with reality, we settle for near-perfect health. And when we die, we are lucky if we leave the world as healthy corpses.

SNOOZE NOT BOOZE

Short of being perfectly healthy or being just plain perfect, we smoke cannabis. Despite all of society's advisories against smoking, we still puff away. We cannabis smokers may be a minority, but minority status does not make us invisible or criminal. A society that has long condoned the use of alcohol and tobacco only recently has begun to reevaluate its historic censure of cannabis. Misled by prohibitionist politicians in their crusade to suppress the civil rights of cannabis users, much of twentieth-century Western society's official standpoint had been dead wrong.

Tobacco smoke is responsible for one out of every five deaths and the leading cause of preventable death among Americans.[3] The second leading cause of preventable death is obesity thanks to the modern American diet and lifestyle.[4] The third leading cause is alcohol.[5] A scant 11 fluid ounces (330 cc) of pure alcohol can kill you.[6] From a bottle of 100-proof whiskey, meaning 50-percent alcohol, you could die by drinking merely 22 fluid ounces (650 cc). That's less than a traditional "fifth of whiskey." For the individual and society, as the most popular mind-altering drug in the world,[7] booze is also the most toxic.[8]

In comparison, no one has ever died of overdose from smoking cannabis in its herbal form. A lethal dose is virtually unattainable,[9] no matter how hell-bent the smoker. According to one guesstimate, to down a fatal dose you would need to smoke eight hundred joints in one sitting.[10] The knockout punch would be the carbon monoxide not the THC. Despite our present day's increased potencies, the zero-percent death rate from fifty years ago remains zero percent today. No day is long enough for you to smoke enough herb to overdose from it. You would fall fast asleep first. Indeed, some insomniacs smoke before bedtime precisely because it helps them to snooze.

A BIG TIFF OVER A LITTLE PUFF

If you are a recreational cannabis smoker, find consolation in knowing that each joint or pipeful that you smoke translates into one less bottle of booze that you otherwise might have swilled. If you smoke just two or three joints a week, that's a volume equivalent to the tobacco in one cigarette. Society sure has made a big tiff over a little puff!

If you are a medical marijuana patient, take heart knowing that by using an herbal remedy you are sparing your body from all the undesirable side effects of the pharmaceutical drug to which you might otherwise have resorted. A pill whose one-page ad in a magazine requires two pages of warnings and disclosures is seldom worth its many risks, especially with risks such as sedation and addiction. As a medical marijuana patient, you've got one leg up on most drug-dependent North Americans, so thumb your nose at Big Pharma, pat yourself on your back, and light up that joint.

BOTANICAL LIBERATION

In college during the hippie sixties when my classmates and I mused while passing around a joint, we predicted that when our generation matured to become doctors, lawyers, and lawmakers, we would swiftly legalize pot, as though with the wave of a magic wand. We felt confident that legalization was just around the corner, was next up on the legislative agenda, or was sure to appear on the next voter referendum. My generation fumbled with that magic wand for thirty years. Plant liberation was not accomplished by my aging hippie generation's grandstanding alone, but by the older and the younger generations both campaigning in unison.

My generation remembers when potheads were branded pariahs and when cannabis was a gateway drug to jail. Now that many states and several nations have fully legalized cannabis for both medicinal and recreational use, no longer will we be threatened by what had been its single greatest harm, that of criminal prosecution. Drug law reform, long overdue, has spread across the political landscape like wildfire. Any attempt here to summarize the quickly evolving statuses of legal cannabis and of cannabis research would amount to a snapshot taken through a narrow window of a rapidly moving express train. This book has served as your travel passport for a safe journey. Enjoy the ride, and enjoy your smoke.

Smoking cannabis has much to commend when compared to smoking tobacco, drinking alcohol, or popping pills. And yet, smoking cannabis has less to commend compared to breathing fresh air. Whether you seek euphoria or analgesia, not taking any drugs is safer than taking drugs. And not smoking any cannabis is safer than smoking cannabis. But if smoke you must, inspirited with your new knowledge of safer ways to smoke, when you light up you now can also lighten up.

Part II

HEALTH RISKS: THE DOWNSIDE OF GETTING HIGH

Chapter Eleven

Cough It Up!

Putting Lungs on the Line

When smoke gets in your eyes, you can wipe away the tears. By the time your tears have dried, the sting in your eyes may already feel relieved. When smoke gets in your lungs, however, irritation can linger. If you are invincible and never bark a cough or catch a cold, you can skip this chapter. But if you count yourself among the rest of us mere mortals, read on.

WHERE THERE'S SMOKE, THERE'S IRE

While smoking cannabis, you might cough. After repeated and heavy smoking, you might even experience bouts of coughing. Routine and constant exposure can impair your throat's and lungs' resistance to infections from pathogens such as fungi,[1] bacteria, and viruses.[2] This in turn increases your susceptibility to respiratory diseases,[3] including chronic ailments such as coughing, wheezing, and spitting.[4] Its smoke can cause sporadic ailments such as a hoarse voice, sore throat, and labored breathing,[5] plus it is the source of both acute and chronic bronchitis.[6] That holds true for repeated exposure to any smoke—tobacco smoke, burnt toast smoke, campfire smoke, and cannabis smoke.

Studies indicate that those who smoke cannabis infrequently, measured as one joint or less a week, rarely suffer more episodes of respiratory illnesses than people who smoke neither cannabis nor tobacco.[7] Research also indicates that habitual smoking, measured as one joint or more a day, can cause far more cases.[8] Since the 1960s, cannabis researchers have been doing a whole lot of calculating. Yet no doctors or researchers have yet drawn a clearly defined line separating light smoking from heavy or casual smoking from habitual. If you consider yourself a heavy smoker, then you probably are. If you consider yourself a light smoker, it's possible that you aren't.

A blurred and uncharted boundary separates infrequent from frequent smoking, so cannabis crusaders and pot prohibitionists have embraced opposing theories based on the same seemingly conflicting evidence. Both sides of the cannabis debate do share some common ground. Both agree that countless studies have proven that cannabis smoking is not healthful for your lungs. Expressed inversely, both agree that no study has ever shown that either casual or habitual smoking improves the health of your lungs.

While cannabis smoke contains many of the same toxic ingredients found in tobacco smoke,[9] unlike tobacco, cannabis does not cause emphysema,[10] or chronic obstructive pulmonary disease (COPD),[11] or pneumonia.[12] Also unlike tobacco, cannabis smoke does not cause lung cancer.[13] This deserves repeating. Cannabis smoke does not cause lung cancer.[14] Even among long-term heavy smokers, cannabis smoke does not cause lung cancer.[15]

Both sides can probably agree that studies of populations of long-time and frequent cannabis smokers link the practice to few physical ailments other than respiratory, gum, or cardiovascular diseases. (See chapters 9 and 12 for more about those last two ailments.) The good news is that health tips for reducing the incidence of these illnesses were already provided to you in this book in part I. So now let's listen through a stethoscope and examine two common respiratory illnesses as yet unmentioned here, namely colds and flu.

A JOINT DISCUSSION OF THE COLD FACTS

One joint *a week* for a year may pose no bodily problems other than the munchies. If you happen to be skinny like a string bean, the munchies are not even a problem. While weight gain is easy to measure, any increased risk for catching colds or the flu is not. While nonsmokers rarely suffer from a hoarse voice, sore throat, labored breathing, wheezing, bronchitis, emphysema, COPD, or lung cancer, nonsmokers do frequently catch colds and come down with the flu. The common cold is so common that it is considered almost normal for nonsmokers of either cannabis or tobacco to catch a cold once a year. That could be why no study has ventured to measure how many more colds per year a cannabis smoker might catch. One study did state that coughing, spitting, and wheezing afflicts approximately one-fifth to one-third of cannabis smokers, but it ventured to offer no figures about colds or flu.[16] One thing we can quantify with certainty, even one cold a year is one too many.

One joint *a day* over the course of many years presents another matter. If that could raise your risk for one or two more colds a year, we're still talking about a lot of maybe "mays" and flaky "ifs" and uncertain "coulds." Such hazy lingo pervades all the medical studies, and that's why as smokers we so often ignore the risks until we actually start sniffling or coughing or wheezing. Regardless of the origins of the colds or flu, when we do get sick, we instinctively know to reduce smoking and to give our overtaxed lungs a rest.

As society's two most widely smoked herbs, the cannabis flower and the tobacco leaf inescapably beg comparison, so let's compare. Except for the cannabinoids in cannabis and the nicotine in tobacco, the two herbs are somewhat similar.[17] As smoke, both pot and cigs contain tar, ash, benzene, phenols, cyanide, aldehydes, nitrogen oxides, carbon monoxide, and a list of other toxic substances with more syllables to their long names than you would want either to pronounce or to inhale.[18]

Puff for puff, cannabis causes less cellular damage to the lungs than does tobacco.[19] At a ratio of around one daily joint of cannabis to one daily pack of cigarettes, even habitual cannabis smokers inhale far fewer puffs than casual tobacco smokers. While inflammation to the lungs is the root cause of these respiratory diseases, cannabinoids reduce inflammation.[20] Call that a consolation prize for smoking cannabis.

Still, cannabis smoke can cause a chronic and dry cough, a protective reflex intended to rid the lungs of irritants. If those irritants get stuck and cause an infection, you could continue trying to cough it up for days. Keep on smoking, and you'll keep on coughing.

SOUNDING THE SMOKE DETECTOR ALARMS

Some past studies have compared daily pot smokers who did not smoke tobacco with people who smoked neither. In part because it was the first, one study is most often cited. Medical records technicians at the Kaiser Permanente Medical Center in Oakland, California, examined the patients' records, not the patients themselves.[21] The researchers compiled data entered for six years from 1979 to 1985, the dark years of pot prohibition when not a lot of potheads openly admitted to their daily consumption of an illegal drug. Tallying cases of sore throats, colds, flu, and bronchitis that were severe enough for patients to seek medical help, the study sought to determine how many more respiratory illnesses the heavy pot smokers suffered compared to the nonsmokers of both pot and tobacco.

When the researchers published their raw data, they dodged the cannabis debate by not formulating any concrete numbers that could be readily understood by the general public. They stated only that "[a]t least one outpatient visit for respiratory problems was made by 36% of the marijuana smokers versus 33% of the nonsmokers."[22] That three-point gap is so insignificant and meaningless that it can hardly imply that smokers get only 3 percent more colds and flu. Peculiarly, patients who consulted their doctors just once for bad colds or flu were tallied with patients who might have visited a dozen times. Which gap is wider? That between one visit and twelve or between one visit and none? Nevertheless, quoting that 3 percent number a statistic favorable for their cause, legalization advocates have often cited those two percentage numbers from this study.[23]

There's more smoke here than meets the nose. Further skewing the numbers, clandestine potheads surely lurked among the cohort of the alleged nonsmokers, yet researchers made no attempt to smoke them out. The brazen stoners who dared to fess up to their flagrant daily violation of drug laws probably lived on the fringes of society and so would have waited longer than nonsmokers to seek medical help. There's no telling how many smokers nursed colds without consulting a doctor. How often do you go running to your doctor when you have only a runny nose?

Even the doctors may have been reluctant to authenticate their patients' use of cannabis. Call me a walking anecdote. In 1991, I implored my doctor to enter into my medical records that I smoked cannabis to suppress the spasms of my spinal cord injury. My doctor declined. In 1992, I again appealed to him. He relented by inscribing an obscure reference to my "inhalation therapy" without actually mentioning cannabis. Many of those doctors during the 1980s whose medical reports were referenced must have been just as resistant. Had my records been included, I would have been counted as a nonsmoker. The flaws of the Kaiser report may be symptomatic of other studies conducted during pot prohibition. It would have long ago been filed away in the dustbin of medical history had not cannabis crusaders seized upon it to further their cause of drug law reform.

Reform indeed has been achieved. The tide has turned in the War on (Some) Drugs. We smokers can now freely confess to our doctors the true extent of our use of cannabis. Studies conducted during our own century, and even better in our own decade, thus provide a clearer picture of how smoking cannabis affects lung health. Study after study has shown how fragile a lung can be when exposed to cannabis smoke. Studies are so numerous that many studies study just the studies. Those are called "systematic studies." One systematic study even studied only other systematic studies.[24] In fact, most of the studies cited in this chapter are systematic studies.

TAKING A BREATHER

Checkmark all that may apply to you. Constant episodes of coughing, wheezing, or spitting? Or recurring cases of sore throat, colds, or flu? Or the rare but unforgettable whammy of bronchitis? How many of these lung busters has set off your alarms?

Smoke a little, and you'll suffer no ill consequences. Smoke a little more, and you might begin to wheeze and cough. Coughing while smoking? Then you've just smoked too much. Coughing after smoking? Then you've been smoking too often. Smoke too much and too often, and you just might memorialize into a medical statistic your downtime laid up with a cold or the flu. No surprise that "flu season" is associated with winter months. Heated indoor air is less humid in winter months, so our nasal passages are drier when indoors, making us more vulnerable to infection. Add smoke into the brew, and your nasal passages become desert dry and all the more vulnerable.

You can breathe a sigh of relief knowing that temporary lung damage linked to cannabis smoke can be remedied simply by greatly reducing your intake or by taking a break altogether. It's always good to take a breather, especially when it comes to breathing.

With its growing legal and social acceptance, more of us will be smoking cannabis, and some of us will be smoking more of it. If we overburden our body's defenses, will we then catch a cold? Predicting illness is an uncertain science, if it is a science at all. One point in our favor is that today's cultivators have been developing strains that are more potent than ever before, for instance 36 percent THC, with more on the way. Even if we smoke cannabis more often, still we can smoke less each time. Even if you seldom smoke and you seldom catch a cold, you now know the preventative steps to take so that if you do catch a cold it is unlikely that its cause was your smoking.

Chapter Twelve

Heartbreaking News
Elevated Blood Pressure and Heartbeat

While you are smoking cannabis, your respiratory system undergoes noticeable stress, signaled by that cough that tumbles out your mouth and rumbles in your ears. But because a heartbeat does not announce itself as loudly as a cough, you might not know that smoking also affects your cardiovascular system, namely your blood vessels and your heart.

THE RISE AND THE FALL

Smoking anything, be it cannabis or tobacco or oregano or banana peels, will cause your heartbeat and your blood pressure to react, usually by rising. Cannabis briefly raises those two vital signs slightly more than does tobacco because, even when consumed by means other than smoking, cannabis generally,[1] and THC specifically,[2] can stress the cardiovascular system. That system reacts in ways that can be unpredictable and, as if it had a mind of its own, illogical. If you wish to take extra precaution, you can always imbibe cannabis through the digestive system, because the stomach absorbs THC more slowly than do the lungs. Otherwise, by simultaneously stirring both smoke and THC into the same cauldron, you can stir up some double trouble.

If you are youthful, slender, and fit, your changes in heartbeat and blood pressure (BP) while you smoke and for an hour after you smoke will hardly be more intense or longer lasting than their surges from strenuous exercise. Such exercise is universally recognized as good for the heart. If smoking indeed puts less strain on your heart than does exercise, you have no need to give a hoot about slight upswings or downturns from smoking. Plus, you can take some comfort knowing that though smoking cannabis raises your heartbeat within minutes of use,[3] that rise is greatest only during the first twenty minutes after smoking,[4] and lasts for no more than two hours.[5] So two hours after smoking cannabis, you can breathe a sigh of relief.

But what if you are mostly sedentary, grossly overweight, and seldom exercise? You would be better off by not even reading this. You would benefit more if you got off your duff and went for a walk in a park. Still reading? If you have a history of strokes or blood clots or cardiac arrest, or if your weak ticker has been diagnosed as a ticking time bomb,[6] or if your high systolic BP (but not high diastolic BP) remains untreated,[7] these already risky health conditions might briefly be complicated by smoking. To exercise caution, you might consider waving a tearful goodbye to vaping or smoking cannabis.

Dangerously high BP can be due to a host of serious medical conditions, of which one is a weak heart. No surprise that high BP is linked to higher risk of heart attack or stroke. Such strokes of bad luck usually befall older adults. Regardless of age, what are the long-term implications of smoking?

Studies rarely agree on how to delineate between young and old adults, and between light and heavy smoking. In one review study of cannabis smokers younger than age forty-four, casual smoking was defined as imbibing less than once every four days, while frequent smoking was defined as more than once a day. For smokers with already high BP, the incidence of stroke over the course of their lives was found to rise slightly, and to rise only slightly more for frequent smokers than for casual smokers.[8] Another review study that drew the line between young and old at fifty years defined light use as less than once a week, while heavy use was more than once a week. It concluded that elevated risk of stroke or heart attack was associated only with heavy smoking not with light smoking.[9]

It's important to remember that such stroke or heart attack did not necessarily occur while or just after smoking. In fact, any immediate danger of stroke or heart attack has been ruled out.[10] Equally ruled out due to a history of smoking cannabis is any higher death rate from stroke or heart attack.[11] The higher risk is associated simply with the odds of suffering a stroke or heart attack over the course of a lifetime. For seasoned smokers, BP rises only slightly or not at all during that first hour after smoking. Longtime and heavy tokers develop a tolerance to that short-term rise.[12] Paradoxically, the BP in some longtime and heavy tokers may even drop while smoking.[13]

This confounding conundrum either wrapped in a joint or stuffed into a pipe gets even more confusing. When longtime heavy smokers abruptly quit and stay clean for weeks or months, their BP goes into catchup mode. It rises and stays up for days or weeks.[14] Science provides no clear explanation, but I offer one theory. If cannabis relieves anxiety for some users, and if their anxiety returns when they abstain from cannabis, then their heightened levels of anxiety may increase their stress, and stress raises BP.

To further complicate matters, posture plays a role. If you stand tall while smoking, your BP might drop a bit. If more typically you sit down while smoking, more likely it will rise. Little wonder that health experts are all over the medical charts on this. Most warn that your BP will rise, while research shows that for some people it could fall. Researchers have even pondered the possibility of applying cannabinoids to lower the BP in those whose preexisting BP was high.[15] If the effects on BP from smoking cannabis may vary either up or down, cliché though it may be, your own mileage will vary. If your BP can fluctuate either way, then your confusion over this medical muddle just might be enough to stress you out. And stress is sure to make your blood pressure rise, not fall.

A DIZZYING EXPERIENCE

If you want to put your own BP to a test, try smoking while leaning back and sitting on your duff, then quickly lurch forward, jump up, and reach for the stars. The abrupt changes in position and posture can make your BP drop very quickly.[16] That in turn might make you feel dizzy.[17] It might even make you faint.[18] Until an esteemed cannabis researcher attested that this once happened to him,[19] I never heard of this happening to anyone outside of the narrow and remote realm of medical studies.

Know that danger lurks not when you pass out, but when you hit the ground. If your life is so boring that you seek the thrill of taking risks and so want to put this exercise to a test, perform it seated in the center of a king size bed. Otherwise, if you faint, rather than knock some sense into your thick skull, you more likely will injure yourself. If you're not bored but are fainthearted, worry in itself can make your BP rise. So if you're worried about fainting by standing up immediately after smoking, either don't stand up or don't smoke cannabis.

As a health-conscious reader, you may already own a blood pressure monitor. If not, consider buying one. Lower-priced digital models render notoriously inaccurate readings of your baseline, but they can give you a fair idea of your surges or drops. Digital models also measure heartbeat, and accurately at that. As if by inherent design, rising or falling heartbeat just happens to be another health risk from smoking cannabis.

THE HEART OF THE MATTER

While you might choose to remain upbeat if smoking only barely elevates your blood pressure, you might have reason to be downbeat about your heartbeat. Blood pressure and heartbeat are connected because arteries and veins are connected to the heart, but the two do not always rise and fall in unison. Same as fickle BP, soon after smoking your heart usually beats faster, though extremely high dosages of cannabis can make it thump slower, and regular use of moderate dosages can induce tolerance prompting no change in heartrate at all.[20]

A healthy heartrate at rest ranges from sixty to one hundred beats per minute (BPM). High heartbeat is measured as more than one hundred BPM.[21] Even in healthy and vibrant young athletes, cannabis usually increases the heartbeat during the first hour after smoking. The peaks documented by medical researchers vary widely. One study calculated average upswings of only 17 percent,[22] which may translate into approximately ten more BPM. Another study calculated an average of twenty to thirty additional BPM. Though the test subjects were seated on their duffs and moved only their hands to lift a joint or a pipe to their lips, that study recorded an upsurge that flew off the charts at forty-four extra beats.[23] Could that meteoric rise have causes other than just cannabis?

Keep in mind that all these studies likely took place in sterile environments of laboratories or hospitals where test subjects were smoking a forbidden drug that during the prohibition era was deemed illegal outside of the lab. Along with the disinfectant, paranoia probably hung in the air. The studies were conducted by medical professionals dressed in bleached white coats. Readings of vital signs that climb higher in doctors' offices than at home are attributed to what is called the "white-coat syndrome." A black-mustached and white-coated Dr. Frankenstein breathing down your neck could spook even the most coldhearted human guinea pig. Or, quite the opposite, the close proximity of a cute young nurse could arouse the passions of some horny macho male. The stirrings of both fear and lust can raise your heartrate.

Better to keep score in the comfort of your home. Conduct some animal experiments, the animal being you. Your own vital signs will not likely hit the heights of the aforementioned high stats, especially if you are an experienced smoker. If you do not own a blood pressure monitor, you probably have a watch conveniently ticking away on your wrist or a clock blinking away on the cellphone resting near your hand. Either location is exactly where you need it to count your heartbeat.

Animal Experiment – Phase 1 – Exercising
Measure and record your heartbeat at rest for one minute. (If you have a blood pressure monitor, measure also your BP.) Then engage in a twenty-minute burst of chest-heaving, breath-panting, sweat-pouring, full-body exercise. When you're ready for your deserved break, take your pulse (and measure your BP). Subtract your resting pulse from your workout pulse and jot down the climb in your BPM. (Do the same for both the top and bottom numbers of your BP.)

In my case, after repeated experiments, there was an insignificant rise in my vital signs but a rise nonetheless. My example is just a wimpy anecdote aspiring to become hard data. The important question is, how much of a rise in yours?

Animal Experiment – Phase 2 – Smoking
Remaining seated for both, measure and record your BPM (and BP) both at rest before smoking and immediately after smoking. Smoke in your typical manner and leisurely spend twenty minutes taking ten tokes. After taking tokes, then take notes, noting the difference.

In my case, and again after repeated self-sacrificing experiments, there was not much difference among my vital signs from smoking. Actually, less from smoking than from exercising. I became high, but my BP and BPM hardly so.

If you clocked in astronomically higher surges, maybe frightening enough to make your heart skip a beat, you should be concerned about both your health and your smoking. Or you might consider that you've been smoking cannabis in an unhealthful way, thus providing you with added incentive to put into action all the health tips of part I of this book.

Despite all the ambiguity postulated in this chapter, one thing is certain. Cannabis produces many beneficial medicinal effects, but it is unlikely that smoking it will benefit either your lungs or your heart.

Notes

FOREWORD

1. Meng Ren, Zihua Tang, Xinhua Wu, Robert Spengler, Hongen Jiang, Yimin Yang, and Nicole Boivin, "The Origins of Cannabis Smoking: Chemical Residue Evidence from the First Millennium BCE in the Pamirs," *Science Advances* 5, no. 6 (June 12, 2019): eaaw1391, https://doi.org/10.1126/sciadv.aaw1391.

ACKNOWLEDGMENTS

1. Dale Gieringer, "Health Tips for Pot Smokers," in *Health Tips for Marijuana Smokers,* ed. Dale Gieringer (San Francisco: California NORML, 1994): 20–23.

2. Mark Mathew Braunstein, "A Connecticut Paraplegic Tells His Story: Marijuana Has Worked the Best in Easing Pain," *The Hartford Courant,* January 12, 1997, Sunday editorials section, C1, C4.

3. Mark Mathew Braunstein, "Getting High and Staying Healthy: How to Reduce the Health Risks of Smoking Marijuana," *Treating Yourself: The Alternative Medicine Journal* 13 (Fall 2008): 55–64, http://treatingyourself.com/magazine/issue13.pdf.

4. Mark Mathew Braunstein, "First Aid for Cannabis Smokers: 10 Ways to Reduce the Health Risks of Smoking Marijuana," *Spirit of Change Magazine: Holistic New England* 29, no. 1 (Spring/Summer 2016): 22–27, http://www.SpiritofChange.org/Spring-2016/First-Aid-for-Cannabis-Smokers.

INTRODUCTION

1. Gillian L. Schauer, Brian A. King, Rebecca E. Bunnell, Gabbi Promoff, and Timothy A. McAfee, "Toking, Vaping, and Eating for Health or Fun: Marijuana Use Patterns in Adults, U.S., 2014," *American Journal of Preventive Medicine* 50, no. 1 (January 2016): 3, http://doi.org/10.1016/j.amepre.2015.05.027.

2. Sarah A. Okey and Madeline H. Meier. "A Within-Person Comparison of the Subjective Effects of Higher vs. Lower-Potency Cannabis," *Drug and Alcohol Dependence* 216, article 108225 (November 2020): 1, https://doi.org/10.1016/j.drugalcdep.2020.108225.

CHAPTER ONE

1. Donald P. Tashkin, "Smoked Marijuana as a Cause of Lung Injury," *Monaldi Archives for Chest Disease* 63, no. 2 (June 2005): 93, https://doi.org/10.4081/monaldi.2005.645, with full text at https://www.monaldi-archives.org/index.php/macd/article/view/645/633.

2. Olivia B. Waxman, "Bill Clinton Said He 'Didn't Inhale' 25 Years Ago," *Time Magazine*, March 29, 2017, https://time.com/4711887/bill-clinton-didnt-inhale-marijuana-anniversary/.

3. James P. Zacny and L. D. Chait, "Breathhold Duration and Response to Marijuana Smoke," *Pharmacology Biochemistry and Behavior* 33, no. 2 (June 1989): 481, https://doi.org/10.1016/0091-3057(89)90534-0.

4. National Academies of Sciences, Engineering, and Medicine, *The Health Effects of Cannabis and Cannabinoids: The Current State of Evidence and Recommendations for Research* (Washington, DC: National Academies Press, 2017): 196, https://doi.org/10.17226/24625.

5. Zacny and Chait, "Breathhold Duration and Response to Marijuana Smoke," 481.

6. James P. Zacny and L. D. Chait, "Response to Marijuana as a Function of Potency and Breathhold Duration," *Psychopharmacology* 103, no. 2 (February 1991): 223, https://doi.org/10.1007/BF02244207.

7. Robert I. Block, Roxanna Farinpour, and Kathleen Braverman, "Acute Effects of Marijuana on Cognition: Relationships to Chronic Effects and Smoking Techniques," *Pharmacology Biochemistry and Behavior* 43, no. 3 (November 1992): 907, https://doi.org/10.1016/0091-3057(92)90424-E.

8. J. L. Azorlosa, M. K. Greenwald, and M. L. Stitzer, "Marijuana Smoking: Effects of Varying Puff Volume and Breathhold Duration," *The Journal*

of Pharmacology and Experimental Therapeutics 272, no. 2 (February 1995): 560, https://www.ncbi.nlm.nih.gov/pubmed/7853169.

9. Mitch Earleywine, *Understanding Marijuana: A New Look at the Scientific Evidence* (Oxford: Oxford University Press, 2002), 157–58.

10. Mitch Earleywine, "Pulmonary Harm and Vaporizers," in *The Pot Book: A Complete Guide to Cannabis*, ed. Julie Holland (Rochester, VT: Park Street Press, 2010), 159.

11. Block et al., "Acute Effects of Marijuana," 907.

12. Earleywine, "Pulmonary Harm and Vaporizers," 159.

CHAPTER TWO

1. CDC (U.S. Centers for Disease Control and Prevention), *How Tobacco Smoke Causes Disease: The Biology and Behavioral Basis for Smoking-Attributable Disease,* Chapter 3, "Chemistry and Toxicology of Cigarette Smoke and Biomarkers of Exposure and Harm" (Atlanta, GA: Centers for Disease Control and Prevention, 2010), 44, https://www.ncbi.nlm.nih.gov/books/NBK53014/.

2. National Academies of Sciences, Engineering, and Medicine, *Acute Exposure Guideline Levels for Selected Airborne Chemicals: Volume 12*, Chapter 1, "Butane" (Washington, DC: National Academies Press, 2012), 17, https://doi.org/10.17226/13377.

3. National Academies, *Acute Exposure Guideline Levels*, 19.

4. Marco Derudi, Simone Gelosa, Andrea Sliepcevich, Andrea Cattaneo, Domenico Cavallo, Renato Rota, and Giuseppe Nano, "Emission of Air Pollutants from Burning Candles with Different Composition in Indoor Environments," *Environmental Science and Pollution Research* 21, no. 6 (March 2014): 4320, https://doi.org/10.1007/s11356-013-2394-2, with full text at https://pubag.nal.usda.gov/catalog/624766.

5. Santino Orecchio, "Polycyclic Aromatic Hydrocarbons (PAHs) in Indoor Emission from Decorative Candles," *Atmospheric Environment* 45, no. 10 (March 2011): 1888, https://doi.org/10.1016/j.atmosenv.2010.12.024.

6. Orecchio, "Polycyclic Aromatic Hydrocarbons," 1895.

7. Amy Westervelt, "Chemical Enemy Number One: How Bad Are Phthalates Really?," *The Guardian*, February 10, 2015, http://www.theguardian.com/lifeandstyle/2015/feb/10/phthalates-plastics-chemicals-research-analysis.

8. Derudi et al., "Emission of Air Pollutants from Burning Candles," 4320.

9. Marco Derudi, Simone Gelosa, Andrea Sliepcevich, Andrea Cattaneo, Domenico Cavallo, Renato Rota, and Giuseppe Nano, "Emissions of Air Pollutants from Scented Candles Burning in a Test Chamber," *Atmospheric*

Environment 55 (August 2012): 257, https://doi.org/10.1016/j.atmosenv.2012.03.027.

10. Philip M. Fine, Glen R. Cass, and Bernd R. T. Simoneit, "Characterization of Fine Particle Emissions from Burning Church Candles," *Environmental Science & Technology* 33, no. 14 (July 1999): 2360, https://doi.org/10.1021/es981039v, with full text at http://lib3.dss.go.th/fulltext/Journal/Environ%20Sci.%20Technology1998-2001/1999/no.14/14,1999%20vol.33,no14,p.2352-2362.pdf.

11. Tunga Salthammer, Jianwei Gu, Sebastian Wientzek, Rob Harrington, and Stefan Thomann, "Measurement and Evaluation of Gaseous and Particulate Emissions from Burning Scented and Unscented Candles," *Environment International* 155 (October 2021): 2–3, https://doi.org/10.1016/j.envint.2021.106590.

12. Salthammer et al., "Measurement and Evaluation," 11.

13. Salthammer et al., "Measurement and Evaluation," 9.

14. Shirley J. Wasson, Zhishi Guo, Jenia A. McBrian, and Laura O. Beach, "Lead in Candle Emissions," *Science of the Total Environment* 296, no. 1–3 (September 2002): 163, https://doi.org/10.1016/S0048-9697(02)00072-4.

15. Wasson et al., "Lead in Candle Emissions," 159.

16. Fine et al., "Characterization of Fine Particle Emissions," 2361.

CHAPTER THREE

1. Gillian L. Schauer, Brian A. King, Rebecca E. Bunnell, Gabbi Promoff, and Timothy A. McAfee, "Toking, Vaping, and Eating for Health or Fun: Marijuana Use Patterns in Adults, U.S., 2014," *American Journal of Preventive Medicine* 50, no. 1 (January 2016): 1, http://doi.org/10.1016/j.amepre.2015.05.027.

2. Andy Geller, "Feds' Joint Effort May OK Weed as Rx for Ill," *New York Post*, March 18, 1999, https://nypost.com/1999/03/18/feds-j0int-effort-may-0k-weed-as-rx-f0r-ill.

3. National Academies of Sciences, Engineering, and Medicine, *Marijuana and Medicine: Assessing the Science Base* (Washington, DC: National Academies Press, 1999), 126, https://doi.org/10.17226/6376.

4. Adrian V., "Why Should You Avoid Bleached Rolling Papers?" May 7, 2017, Everyone Does It (website) accessed July 5, 2021, https://www.everyonedoesit.com/blogs/blog/why-should-you-avoid-bleached-rolling-papers.

5. Anthony Franciosi, "Rolling Papers: The Ultimate Guide," Honest Marijuana Company (website) accessed July 5, 2021, https://honestmarijuana.com/rolling-papers/.

6. John J. Mariani, Daniel Brooks, Margaret Haney, and Frances R. Levin, "Quantification and Comparison of Marijuana Smoking Practices: Blunts, Joints, and Pipes," *Drug and Alcohol Dependence* 113, no. 2-3 (January 15, 2011): 250, https://doi.org/10.1016/j.drugalcdep.2010.08.008.

7. LaTrice Montgomery, Erin A. McClure, Rachel L. Tomko, Susan C. Sonne, Theresa Winhusen, Garth E. Terry, Jason T. Grossman, and Kevin M. Gray, "Blunts versus Joints: Cannabis Use Characteristics and Consequences among Treatment-Seeking Adults," *Drug and Alcohol Dependence* 198 (May 2019): 109, https://doi.org/10.1016/j.drugalcdep.2019.01.041.

8. CDC (Centers for Disease Control and Prevention), *How Tobacco Smoke Causes Disease: The Biology and Behavioral Basis for Smoking-Attributable Disease,* Chapter 3, "Chemistry and Toxicology of Cigarette Smoke and Biomarkers of Exposure and Harm" (Atlanta, GA: Centers for Disease Control and Prevention, 2010), 44, https://www.ncbi.nlm.nih.gov/books/NBK53014/.

9. FDA (U.S. Food and Drug Administration), "Applications for Premarket Review of New Tobacco Products," http://www.fda.gov/files/tobacco%20products/published/PDF-Ver_Draft-Guidance-for-Industry-Applications-for-Premarket-Review-of-New-Tobacco-Products.pdf.

10. SC Labs (Science of Cannabis Laboratories), "Rolling Papers Tested for Heavy Metals and Pesticides," (September, 2, 2020): 4, http://www.sclabs.com/wp-content/uploads/2020/09/SC-Labs-Report_Rolling_Papers_MKT00308.pdf.

11. SC Labs, "Rolling Papers Tested," 6.

12. Hidemi Ito, Keitaro Matsuo, Hideo Tanaka, Devin C. Koestler, Hernando Ombao, John Fulton, Akiko Shibata, Manabu Fujita, Hiromi Sugiyama, Midori Soda, Tomotaka Sobue, and Vincent Mor, "Nonfilter and Filter Cigarette Consumption and the Incidence of Lung Cancer by Histological Type in Japan and the United States: Analysis of 30-Year Data from Population-Based Cancer Registries," *International Journal of Cancer* 128, no. 8 (April 15, 2011): 1925, https://doi.org/10.1002/ijc.25531.

13. Tik Root, "Cigarette Butts Are Toxic Plastic Pollution. Should They be Banned?," August 9, 2019, *National Geographic* (website) accessed July 5, 2019, https://www.nationalgeographic.com/environment/article/cigarettes-story-of-plastic.

14. Root, "Cigarette Butts Are Toxic Plastic Pollution."

15. Bradford Harris, "The Intractable Cigarette 'Filter Problem,'" *Tobacco Control* 20, no. 1 (April 18, 2011): i10, https://doi.org/10.1136%2Ftc.2010.040113.

16. Ito et al., "Nonfilter and Filter Cigarette Consumption, 1926–27.

17. J. Rimington, "The Effect of Filters on the Incidence of Lung Cancer in Cigarette Smokers," *Environmental Research* 24, no. 1 (February 1981): 162, https://doi.org/10.1016/0013-9351(81)90142-0.

18. Rick Doblin, "The MAPS / California NORML Water Pipe Study," *Newsletter of the Multidisciplinary Association of Psychedelic Studies* (MAPS) 5, no. 1 (Summer 1994), https://maps.org/news-letters/v05n1/05119wps.html.

19. "Cannabis Research," Bedrocan International (website) accessed July 12, 2021, https://bedrocan.com/medicinal-cannabis/cannabis-research/.

20. Frank van der Kooy, B. Pomahacova, and R.Verpoorte, "Cannabis Smoke Condensate I: The Effect of Different Preparation Methods on Tetrahydrocannabinol Levels," *Inhalation Toxicology: International Forum for Respiratory Health* 20, no. 9 (November 2008): 804, http://doi.org/10.1080/08958370802013559 and full text at https://bedrocan.com/wp-content/uploads/2008a-cannabis-smoke-condensate-i-the-effect-of-different-preparation-methods-on-tetrahydrocannabinol-levels_van-der-kooy.pdf.

CHAPTER FOUR

1. Cynthia Kuhn, Scott Swartzwelder, and Wilkie Wilson, *Buzzed: The Straight Facts about the Most Used and Abused Drugs from Alcohol to Ecstasy*, second ed. (New York: W.W. Norton, 2003), 140.

2. Mario Perez-Reyes, "Marijuana Smoking: Factors That Influence the Bioavailability of Tetrahydrocannabinol," *Research Findings on Smoking of Abused Substances, NIDA Research Monograph* 99 (1990): 60, http://citeseerx.ist.psu.edu/viewdoc/summary?doi=10.1.1.517.3186.

3. Michael Backes, *Cannabis Pharmacy: A Practical Guide to Medical Marijuana* (New York: Black Dog & Leventhal Publishers, 2014), 150.

4. Rick Doblin, "The MAPS / California NORML Water Pipe Study," *Newsletter of the Multidisciplinary Association of Psychedelic Studies* (MAPS) 5, no. 1 (Summer 1994), https://maps.org/news-letters/v05n1/05119wps.html.

5. Nicolas Lau, Paloma Sales, Sheigla Averill, Fiona Murphy, Sye-Ok Sato, and Sheigla Murphy, "Responsible and Controlled Use: Older Cannabis Users and Harm Reduction," *International Journal of Drug Policy* 26, no. 8 (August 2015): 710, https://doi.org/10.1016/j.drugpo.2015.03.008, with full text at https://www.ncbi.nlm.nih.gov/pmc/articles/PMC4499492.

CHAPTER FIVE

1. Nicholas V. Cozzi, "Effects on Water Filtration on Marijuana Smoke: A Literature Review," *Newsletter of the Multidisciplinary Association for Psychedelic Studies (MAPS)* 4, no. 2 (1993), http://www.ukcia.org/research/EffectsOfWaterFiltrationOnMarijuanaSmoke.php.

2. Peter Stafford, *Psychedelics Encyclopedia*, third ed. (Berkeley, CA: Ronin Publishing, 1992), 221.

3. Stafford, *Psychedelics Encyclopedia*, 221.

4. Andrew Weil and Winifred Rosen, *From Chocolate to Morphine: Everything You Need to Know about Mind-Altering Drugs*, revised ed. (Boston: Houghton Mifflin, 2004), 78.

5. Robert Ross MacLean, Gerald W. Valentine, Peter I. Jatlow, and Mehmet Sofuoglu, "Inhalation of Alcohol Vapor: Measurement and Implications," *Alcoholism: Clinical and Experimental Research* 41, no. 2 (February 2017): 240, https://doi.org/10.1111/acer.13291, with full text at https://www.ncbi.nlm.nih.gov/pmc/articles/PMC6143144/.

6. Cozzi, "Effects on Water Filtration."

7. Dale Gieringer, "Marijuana Water Pipe and Vaporizer Study," *Newsletter of the Multidisciplinary Association for Psychedelic Studies (MAPS)* 6, no. 3 (Summer 1996), https://maps.org/news-letters/v06n3/06359mj1.html.

8. Ed Rosenthal, Dale Gieringer, and Tod Mikuriya, *Medical Marijuana Handbook: A Guide to Therapeutic Use* (Oakland, CA: Quick American Archives, 1997), 107.

9. Nicolas Lau, Paloma Sales, Sheigla Averill, Fiona Murphy, Sye-Ok Sato, and Sheigla Murphy, "Responsible and Controlled Use: Older Cannabis Users and Harm Reduction," *International Journal of Drug Policy* 26, no. 8 (August 2015): 710, https://doi.org/10.1016/j.drugpo.2015.03.008.

10. W. J. Munckhof, A. Konstantinos, M. Wamsley, M. Mortlock, and C. Gilpin, "A Cluster of Tuberculosis Associated with Use of a Marijuana Water Pipe," *The International Journal of Tuberculosis and Lung Diseases* 7, no. 9 (September 1, 2003): 864, http//:www.ingentaconnect.com/content/iuatld/ijtld/2003/00000007/00000009/art00009#.

11. John E. Oeltmann, Eyal Oren, Maryam B. Haddad, Linda K. Lake, Theresa A. Harrington, Kashef Ijaz, and Masahiro Narita, "Tuberculosis Outbreak in Marijuana Users, Seattle, Washington, 2004," *Emerging Infectious Diseases* 12, no. 7 (July 2006): 1157, https://doi.org/10.3201/eid1207.051436.

CHAPTER SIX

1. Ali J. Zarrabi, Jennifer K. Frediani, and Joshua M. Levy, "The State of Cannabis Research Legislation in 2020," *New England Journal of Medicine* 382, no. 20 (May 2020): 1876–77, https://doi.org/10.1056/NEJMp2003095, with full text at https://www.ncbi.nlm.nih.gov/pmc/articles/PMC7302267/.

2. Nicholas Chadi, Claudia Minato, and Richard Stanwick, "Cannabis Vaping: Understanding the Health Risks of a Rapidly Emerging Trend,"

Paediatrics & Child Health 25, no. 1 (June 2020): S17, https://doi.org/10.1093 /pch/pxaa016.

3. Dharma N. Bhatta and Stanton A. Glantz, "Association of E-Cigarette Use with Respiratory Disease among Adults: A Longitudinal Analysis," *American Journal of Preventive Medicine* 58, no. 2 (February 2020): 189, https://doi .org/10.1016/j.amepre.2019.07.028.

4. Nate Seltenrich, "Cannabis Contaminants: Regulating Solvents, Microbes, and Metals in Legal Weed," *Environmental Health Perspectives* 127, no.8 (August 2019): 4–5, https://doi.org/10.1289/EHP5785.

5. Seltenrich, "Cannabis Contaminants," 4.

6. Eric Lindblom, "Marijuana and Vaping: Shadowy Past, Dangerous Present," *The New York Times*, October 21, 2019, https://www.nytimes.com /2019/10/21/health/marijuana-and-vaping-shadowy-past-dangerous-present .html.

7. ATSDR (Agency for Toxic Substances and Disease Registry, U.S. Centers for Disease Control and Prevention), "Public Health Statement for Propylene Glycol," CAS#57-55-6 (September 1997): 3, https://www.atsdr.cdc.gov /toxprofiles/tp189-c1-b.pdf.

8. FDA (U.S. Food and Drug Administration), "Harmful and Potentially Harmful Constituents in Tobacco Products; Established List; Proposed Additions," *Federal Register* 84, no. 150, Docket No. FDA-N-0143 (August 5, 2019): 38034, https://www.govinfo.gov/content/pkg/FR-2019-08-05/pdf/2019 -16658.pdf.

9. Dale Gieringer, "Marijuana Water Pipe and Vaporizer Study," *Newsletter of the Multidisciplinary Association for Psychedelic Studies (MAPS)* 6, no. 3 (Spring 1996), https://www.ojp.gov/library/abstracts/waterpipe-study, with full text at https://maps.org/news-letters/v06n3/06359mj1.html.

10. Dale H. Gieringer, "Cannabis 'Vaporization': A Promising Strategy for Smoke Harm Reduction," *Journal of Cannabis Therapeutics* 1, no. 3–4 (2001): 164–66, https://www.cannabis-med.org/data/pdf/2001-03-04-9.pdf.

11. Dale Gieringer, Joseph St. Laurent, and Scott Goodrich, "Cannabis Vaporizer Combines Efficient Delivery of THC with Effective Suppression of Pyrolytic Compounds," *Journal of Cannabis Therapeutics* 4, no. 1 (February 26, 2004): 9, https://doi.org/10.1300/J175v04n01_02, with full text at https:// www.ukcia.org/research/CannabisVaporizer.pdf.

12. Gieringer et al., "Cannabis Vaporizer," 15.

13. Lindblom, "Marijuana and Vaping: Shadowy Past, Dangerous Present."

14. Gieringer et al., "Cannabis Vaporizer," 22.

15. Donald I. Abrams, H. P. Vizoso, S. B. Shade, C. Jay, M. E. Kelly, and N. L. Benowitz, "Vaporization as a Smokeless Cannabis Delivery System: A Pilot Study," *Clinical Pharmacology & Therapeutics* 82, no. 5 (November 2007):

573, https://doi.org/10.1038/sj.clpt.6100200, with full text at https://sci-hub .se/10.1038/sj.clpt.6100200.

16. Abrams et al., "Vaporization as a Smokeless Cannabis Delivery System," 576.

17. Abrams et al., "Vaporization as a Smokeless Cannabis Delivery System," 575.

18. Nicholas T. Van Dam and Mitch Earleywine, "Pulmonary Function in Cannabis Users. Support for a Clinical Trial of the Vaporizer," *International Journal of Drug Policy* 21, No.6 (November 2010): 512, https:// doi.org/10.1016/j.drugpo.2010.04.001, with full text at https://www.albany .edu/~me888931/Vaporizer.pdf.

19. Mitch Earleywine and Sara Smucker Barnwell, "Decreased Respiratory Symptoms in Cannabis Users Who Vaporize," *Harm Reduction Journal* 4, no. 11 (2007): 2, https://doi.org/10.1186/1477-7517-4-11.

20. Tory R. Spindle, Edward J. Cone, Nicolas J. Schlienz, John M. Mitchell, George E. Bigelow, Ronald Flegel, Eugene Hayes, and Ryan Vandrey, "Acute Effects of Smoked and Vaporized Cannabis in Healthy Adults Who Infrequently Use Cannabis: A Crossover Trial," *Journal of the American Medical Association (JAMA)* 1, no. 7 (November 30, 2018): 1, https://doi.org/10.1001 /jamanetworkopen.2018.4841.

21. Jeremy Peters and Joseph Chien, "Contemporary Routes of Cannabis Consumption: A Primer for Clinicians," *The Journal of the American Osteopathic Association* 118, no. 2 (February 1, 2018): 67, https://doi.org/10.7556 /jaoa.2018.020.

22. Christian Lanz, Johan Mattsson, Umut Soydaner, and Rudolf Brenneisen, "Medicinal Cannabis: *In Vitro* Validation of Vaporizers for the Smoke-Free Inhalation of Cannabis," *Public Library of Science (PLOS)* 11, no. 1 (January 19, 2016): 4, https://doi.org/10.1371/journal.pone.0147286.

23. Lanz et al., "Medicinal Cannabis," 14.

24. Lanz et al., "Medicinal Cannabis," 1.

25. John M. McPartland and Ethan B. Russo, "Cannabis and Cannabis Extracts: Greater Than the Sum of Their Parts?" *Journal of Cannabis Therapeutics* 1, no. 3–4 (June 2001): 111–14, https://doi.org/10.1300/J175v01n03_08, with full text at http://www.cannabis-med.org/data/pdf/2001-03-04-7.pdf.

26. Earleywine and Smucker Barnwell, "Decreased Respiratory Symptoms," 2–3.

27. Mallory Loflin and Mitch Earleywine, "No Smoke, No Fire: What the Initial Literature Suggests Regarding Vapourized Cannabis and Respiratory Risk," *Canadian Journal of Respiratory Therapy* 51, no. 1 (Winter 2015): 7, https://www.ncbi.nlm.nih.gov/pmc/articles/PMC4456813/.

28. Roger N. Bloor, Tianshu S. Wang, Patrik Španěl, and David Smith, "Ammonia Release from Heated 'Street' Cannabis Leaf and Its Potential Toxic Effects on Cannabis Users," *Addiction* 103, no. 10 (October 2008): 1674–75, https://doi.org/10.1111/j.1360-0443.2008.02281.x.

CHAPTER SEVEN

1. Nicolas Sullivan, Sytze Elzinga, and Jeffrey C. Raber, "Determination of Pesticide Residues in Cannabis Smoke," *Journal of Toxicology* 2013, ID 378168 (May 2013):1, http://dx.doi.org/10.1155/2013/378168.
2. Sullivan et al., "Determination of Pesticide Residues in Cannabis Smoke," 1.
3. Sullivan et al., "Determination of Pesticide Residues in Cannabis Smoke," 6.
4. Jesse Kornbluth, "Poisonous Fallout from the War on Marijuana," *New York Times Magazine*, November 19, 1978, https://www.nytimes.com/1978/11/19/archives/poisonous-fallout-from-the-war-on-marijuana-paraquat.html.
5. Philip J. Landrigan, Kenneth E. Powell, Levy M. James, and Philip R. Taylor, "Paraquat and Marijuana: Epidemiological Risk Assessment," *American Journal of Public Health* 73, no. 7 (July 1983): 784, https://ajph.aphapublications.org/doi/pdf/10.2105/AJPH.73.7.784.
6. Jerome London, "Paraquat Pot: The True Story of How the US Government Tried to Kill Weed Smokers with a Toxic Chemical in the 1980s," *Thought Catalog*, last modified February 4, 2021, https://thoughtcatalog.com/jeremy-london/2018/08/paraquat-pot.
7. Martin Jelsma and Virginia Montañés, "Vicious Circle: The Chemical and Biological 'War on Drugs,'" *Transnational Institute's Drugs and Democracy Programme* (March 2001): 2, https://www.tni.org/files/download/vicious circle-e.pdf.
8. Rafael Lanaro, José L. Costa, Silvia O. S. Cazenave, Luiz A. Zanolli-Filho, Marina F. M. Tavares, and Alice A. M. Chasin, "Determination of Herbicides Paraquat, Glyphosate, and Aminomethylphosphonic Acid [AMPA] in Marijuana Samples by Capillary Electrophoresis," *Journal of Forensic Sciences* 60, no. 1 (January 2015): S241, https://doi.org/10.1111/1556-4029.12628.
9. Jeffrey P. Prestemon, Frank H. Koch, Geoffrey H. Donovan, and Mary T. Lihou, "Cannabis Legalization by States Reduces Illegal Growing on US National Forests," *Ecological Economics* 164, article 106366 (October 2019), https://doi.org/10.1016/j.ecolecon.2019.106366.

10. Nate Seltenrich, "Into the Weeds: Regulating Pesticides in Cannabis," *Environmental Health Perspectives* 127, no. 4 (April 2019): 5, https://doi.org/10.1289/EHP5265.

11. Dave Stone, "Cannabis, Pesticides and Conflicting Laws: The Dilemma for Legalized States and Implications for Public Health," *Regulatory Toxicology and Pharmacology* 69 (2014): 285, http://dx.doi.org/10.1016/j.yrtph.2014.05.015.

12. Bureau of Cannabis Control (BCC) of the California Environmental Protection Agency, Department of Pesticide Regulation (DPR), https://cannabis.ca.gov/cannabis-regulations.

13. Bureau of Cannabis Control (BCC), "Medicinal and Adult-Use Cannabis Regulatory [in some texts called "Regulations"] and Safety Act" (MAUCRSA), https://leginfo.legislature.ca.gov/faces/codes_displayexpanded branch.xhtml?tocCode=BPC&division=10.&title=&part=&chapter=&article =&nodetreepath=14.

14. Bureau of Cannabis Control (BCC), "Cannabis Pesticides That Cannot Be Used," September 2018, https://www.cdpr.ca.gov/docs/cannabis/cannot_use _pesticide.pdf.

15. Seltenrich, "Into the Weeds," 3.

16. Bureau of Cannabis Control (BCC), "Cannabis Batch Testing Certificate of Analysis," January 18, 2019, https://docs.google.com/viewer ?url=https%3A%2F%2Fbcc.ca.gov%2Fclear%2Fdocuments%2Fweekly %2F20190122_update.xlsx.

17. Jay Feldman and Drew Toher, "Pesticide Use in Marijuana Production: Safety Issues and Sustainable Options," *Pesticides and You: A Quarterly Publication of Beyond Pesticides* 34, no. 4 (Winter 2014–15): 19, https://www.beyondpesticides.org/assets/media/documents/watchdog/documents/Pesti cideUseCannabisProduction.pdf.

18. Amelia Taylor and Jason W. Birkett, "Pesticides in Cannabis: A Review of Analytical and Toxicological Considerations," *Drug Testing and Analysis* 12, no. 2 (February 2020): 180, https://doi.org/10.1002/dta.2747.

19. Sanka N. Atapattu and Kevin R. D. Johnson, "Pesticide Analysis in Cannabis Products," *Journal of Chromatography* 1612, article 460656 (February 8, 2020): 2, https://doi.org/10.1016/j.chroma.2019.460656.

20. Atapattu and Johnson, "Pesticide Analysis in Cannabis Products," 2.

21. Sullivan et al., "Determination of Pesticide Residues in Cannabis Smoke," 2.

22. Seltenrich, "Into the Weeds," 3.

23. Los Angeles City Attorney, "City Attorney Explains Medical Marijuana Issue on NBC," Los Angeles City Attorney Blogspot, October 13, 2009, http://lacityorgatty.blogspot.com/2009/10/city-attorney-explains-medical.html.

24. Zackary Montoya, Matthieu Conroy, Brian D. Vanden Heuvel, Christopher S. Pauli, and Sang-Hyuck Park, "Cannabis Contaminants Limit Pharmacological Use of Cannabidiol," *Frontiers in Pharmacology* 11, article 571832 (September 11, 2020): 6, https://doi.org/10.3389/fphar.2020.571832.

25. Pablo Valdes-Donoso, Daniel A. Sumner, and Robin Goldstein, "Costs of Cannabis Testing Compliance: Assessing Mandatory Testing in the California Cannabis Market," *PLOS ONE* 15, no. 4 (April 23, 2020): 15, https://doi.org/10.1371/journal.pone.0232041.

26. Valdes-Donoso et al., "Costs of Cannabis Testing Compliance," 18.

27. Valdes-Donoso et al., "Costs of Cannabis Testing Compliance," 1.

28. Ajay Mishra and Nikhil Dave, "Neem Oil Poisoning: Case Report of an Adult with Toxic Encephalopathy," *Indian Journal of Critical Care* 17, no. 5 (September-October 2013): 322, https://dx.doi.org/10.4103%2F0972-5229.120330.

29. M. H. Kollef, "Adult Respiratory Distress Syndrome after Smoke Inhalation from Burning Poison Ivy," *Journal of the American Medical Association (JAMA)* 274, no. 4 (July 26,1995): 358–59, https://doi.org/10.1001/jama.1995.03530040086059.

30. Emily Earlenbaugh, "Is Neem Oil Causing Cannabinoid Hyperemesis Syndrome?" Leafly, June 24, 2019, https://www.leafly.com/news/health/neem-oil-cannabinoid-hyperemesis-syndrome.

31. J. H. Allen, G. M. de Moore, H. Heddle, and J. C. Twartz, "Cannabinoid Hyperemesis: Cyclical Hyperemesis in Association with Chronic Cannabis Abuse," *Gut* 53, no. 11 (November 2004): 1570, https://doi.org/10.1136/gut.2003.036350.

32. Douglas A. Simonoetto, Amy S. Oxentenko, Margot L. Herman, and Jason H. Szostek, "Cannabinoid Hyperemesis: A Case Series of 98 Patients," *Mayo Clinic Proceedings* 87, no. 2 (February 2012): 118, https://doi.org/10.1016/j.mayocp.2011.10.005.

33. Earlenbaugh, "Is Neem Oil Causing Cannabinoid Hyperemesis Syndrome?"

34. Ethan B. Russo, Chris Spooner, Len May, Ryan Leslie, and Venetia L. Whiteley, "Cannabinoid Hyperemesis Syndrome Survey and Genomic Investigation," *Cannabis and Cannabinoid Research* 10, no. 10 (July 5, 2021): 8, https://doi.org/10.1089/can.2021.0046.

35. Joel Grover and Matthew Glasser, "Pesticides and Pot: What's California Smoking?" NBC-TV Los Angeles, February 22, 2017, https://www.nbclosangeles.com/news/i-team-marijuana-pot-pesticide-california/31341/.

36. Taylor and Birkett, "Pesticides in Cannabis."

37. Grover and Glasser, "Pesticides and Pot."

38. Bureau of Cannabis Control (BCC), "Cannabis Pesticides That Cannot Be Used."

39. Montoya et al., "Cannabis Contaminants Limit Pharmacological Use of Cannabidiol," 6.

40. Nate Seltenrich, "Cannabis Contaminants: Regulating Solvents, Microbes, and Metals in Legal Weed," *Environmental Health Perspectives* 127, no. 8 (August 2019): 3, https://doi.org/10.1289/EHP5785.

41. BCC, "Cannabis Batch Testing Certificate of Analysis."

42. Montoya et al., "Cannabis Contaminants," 4.

43. Mowgli Holmes, John M. Vyas, William Steinbach, and John McPartland, "Microbiological Safety Testing of Cannabis," *Cannabis Safety Institute* (May 2015): 16–17, https://cdn.technologynetworks.com/tn/Resources/pdf/microbiological-safety-testing-of-cannabis.pdf.

44. Montoya et al., "Cannabis Contaminants," 4.

45. Montoya et al., "Cannabis Contaminants," 3.

46. Holmes et al., "Microbiological Safety Testing of Cannabis," 21.

47. Yousef Gargani, Paul Bishop, and David W. Denning, "Too Many Mouldy Joints: Marijuana and Chronic Pulmonary Aspergillosis," *Mediterranean Journal of Hematology and Infectious Diseases* 3, no. 1 (January 13, 2011): 1, http://dx.doi.org/10.4084/MJHID.2011.005.

48. Medicinal Genomics Corporation, "Aspergillus: The Most Dangerous Cannabis Pathogen," Medicinal Genomics, accessed August 20, 2021, https://www.medicinalgenomics.com/aspergillus-dangerous-cannabis-pathogen/.

49. Seltenrich, "Cannabis Contaminants," 3.

50. Medicinal Genomics Corp., "Aspergillus."

51. Holmes et al., "Microbiological Safety Testing of Cannabis," 27.

52. Robert Connell Clarke, *Marijuana Botany: An Advanced Study: The Propagation and Breeding of Distinctive Cannabis* (Berkeley, CA: And/Or Press, 1981), 152.

53. Ed Rosenthal with David Downs, *Marijuana Harvest: How to Maximize Quality and Yield in Your Cannabis Garden* (Piedmont, CA: Quick American Publishing, 2017): 181.

54. Kieran Nicholson, "Denver Marijuana Cultivator Issues Statewide Recall Over High Mold and Yeast Levels," *The Denver Post*, October 14, 2019, https://www.denverpost.com/2019/10/14/denver-marijuana-recall.

55. R. Steve Pappas, "Toxic Elements in Tobacco and in Cigarette Smoke: Inflammation and Sensitization," *Metallomics* 3, no. 11 (November 2011): 1181, https://doi.org/10.1039/c1mt00066g.

56. David V. Gauvin, Zachary J. Zimmermann, Joshua Yoder, and Rachel Tapp, "Marijuana Toxicity: Heavy Metal Exposure through State-Sponsored Access to 'la Fee Verte,'" *Pharmaceutical Regulatory Affairs* 7, no. 1 (April 1, 2018): 5, https://doi.org/10.4172/2167-7689.1000202.

57. Pappas, "Toxic Elements in Tobacco and in Cigarette Smoke," 1187.

58. Seltenrich, "Cannabis Contaminants," 4.

8:a

59. Murad Ali Khan, Abdul Wajid, Suhail Noor, Fareedullah Khan Khattak, Saeed Akhtar, and Inayat Ur Rahman, "Effect of Soil Contamination on Some Heavy Metals Content of Cannabis Sativa," *Journal of the Chemical Society of Pakistan* 30, no. 6 (December 2008): 806. https://jcsp.org.pk/issueDetail.aspx?aid=5d7c3bc9-8cfd-4194-a905-aa1f7a9c324e.

60. Montoya et al., "Cannabis Contaminants," 5.

61. Montoya et al., "Cannabis Contaminants," 5.

62. Franziska P. Busse, Georg Martin Fiedler, Alexander Leichtle, Helmut Hentschel, and Michael Stumvoll, "Lead Poisoning Due to Adulterated Marijuana in Leipzig," *Deutsches Ärzteblatt International* 105, no. 44 (October 2008): 757, https://doi.org/10.3238/arztebl.2008.0757.

63. Khan et al., "Effect of Soil Contamination on Some Heavy Metals Content of Cannabis Sativa," 807.

64. Seltenrich, "Cannabis Contaminants," 4.

65. Montoya et al., "Cannabis Contaminants," 7.

66. Atapattu and Johnson, "Pesticide Analysis in Cannabis Products," 2.

67. Atapattu and Johnson, "Pesticide Analysis in Cannabis Products," 2.

68. Montoya et al., "Cannabis Contaminants," 7.

69. Jessica McKeil, "The Dangers of PGR Weed and How to Identify It," International HighLife, October 25, 2020, https://internationalhighlife.com/the-dangers-of-pgr-weed-and-how-to-identify-it.

70. Clarke, *Marijuana Botany*, 130.

71. McKeil, "The Dangers of PGR Weed."

72. Francis Cassidy, "PGR Weed Is Risky and Here's How to Spot It," RxLeaf, September 24, 2019, https://www.rxleaf.com/dangers-pgr-weed-identify-before-buy-medical-cannabis/.

73. James Jett, Emily Stone, Graham Warren, and K. Michael Cummings, "Cannabis Use, Lung Cancer, and Related Issues," *Journal of Thoracic Oncology* 13, issue 4 (April 1, 2018): 483, https://doi.org/10.1016/j.jtho.2017.12.013.

74. Zuzana Zelinkova and Thomas Wenzl, "The Occurrence of 16 EPA PAHs in Food: A Review," *Polycyclic Aromatic Compounds* 35, no. 2–4 (2015): 250, https://doi.org/10.1080/10406638.2014.918550.

75. Elena Schmidt, "PAH: This Is Why We Test Hemp and Cannabis for Polycyclic Aromatic Hydrocarbons," ACS Laboratory, August 5, 2020, https://acslabcannabis.com/blog/education/pah-this-is-why-we-test-hemp-cannabis-for-polycyclic-aromatic-hydrocarbons/#wild.

76. Bonny K. Larsson, Greger P. Sahlberg, Anders T. Eriksson, and Leif Á. Busk, "Polycyclic Aromatic Hydrocarbons in Grilled Food," *Journal of Agricultural and Food Chemistry* 31, no. 4 (1983): 872, https://pubs.acs.org/doi/pdf/10.1021/jf00118a049?casa_token=0WH6tvcFNWIAAAAA:rJp6gOZEaaRliJ-Zt_lFp7ZNHXeKRbQqgV0MKCPuzvvapA9V6tskoXqqFVzcp8WITqL-aaDL6lBHdiZp.

77. Vasudha Bansal and Ki-Hyun Kim, "Review of PAH Contamination in Food Products and Their Health Hazards," *Environment International* 84 (July 20, 2015): 27, https://doi.org/10.1016/j.envint.2015.06.016.

78. Montoya et al., "Cannabis Contaminants," 7.

79. Schmidt, "PAH."

80. Schmidt, "PAH."

81. Montoya et al., "Cannabis Contaminants," 7.

82. David Migoya and Ricardo Baca, "Hickenlooper Issues Executive Order to Declare Tainted Pot a Threat to Public Safety," *The Denver Post*, October 2, 2016, https://www.denverpost.com/2015/11/12/hickenlooper-issues-executive-order-to-declare-tainted-pot-a-threat-to-public/.

83. David Migoya and Ricardo Baca, "Colorado Yields to Marijuana Industry Pressure on Pesticides," *The Denver Post*, October 3, 2015, https://www.denverpost.com/2015/10/03/colorado-yields-to-marijuana-industry-pressure-on-pesticides/.

84. David Migoya and Ricardo Baca, "Colorado Pot Industry Steps Up Pesticide Fight against Regulators," *The Denver Post*, May 1, 2016, https://www.denverpost.com/2016/05/01/colorado-pot-industry-steps-up-pesticide-fight-against-regulators/.

85. Dana Rubenstein, Amanda Eisenberg, and Nick Niedzwiadek, "De Blasio's Marijuana Dreams Already Facing Headwinds in Albany," Politico, December 20, 2018, https://www.politico.com/states/new-york/albany/story/2018/12/20/de-blasios-marijuana-dreams-already-facing-headwinds-in-albany-761652.

86. Tim Wilson, "The Wild West of Organic Cannabis," StratCann, February 10, 2021, https://stratcann.com/2021/02/10/the-wild-west-of-organic-cannabis/.

87. Anna E. Epperson, Lisa Henriksen, and Judith J. Prochaska, "Natural American Spirit Brand Marketing Casts Health Halo around Smoking," *American Journal of Public Health* 107, no. 5 (May 2017): 669, https://doi.org/10.2105/AJPH.2017.303719, with full text at https://www.ncbi.nlm.nih.gov/pmc/articles/PMC5388969/.

88. California Department of Food and Agriculture (CDFA), CalCannabis Cultivation Licensing, OCal Program, "Introducing the California Department of Food and Agriculture's OCal Program," https://www.cdfa.ca.gov/calcannabis/ocal.html.

89. Clean Green Certified, https://cleangreencertified.com.

90. Oregon Sungrown Farm Certification, https://www.oregonsungrown.org/osg-certification.

91. Cannabis Certification Council's CCC Organically Grown Cannabis Certification, https://cannabiscertificationcouncil.org.

92. Pure Regenerative Cannabis Movement's Pure Certification, http://dempurefarms.com/pure-certification-agreement.

93. Certified Kind, https://www.certified-kind.com/certified-kind-rules.

94. Sun+Earth Certified, https://www.certified-kind.com/sunearth-certified.

95. Cannabis Safety and Quality Certification, https://www.csqcertification .com.

96. Voltaire, *Candide* (New York: Boni & Liveright, 1918): 308, https:// gutenberg.org/ebooks/19942.

CHAPTER EIGHT

1. Yehiel Gaoni and Raphael Mechoulam, "Isolation and Structure of Delta-Tetrahydrocannabinol and Other Neutral Cannabinoids from Hashish," *Journal of American Chemistry* 93, no.1 (January 13, 1971): 217, https://pubs.acs.org /doi/pdf/10.1021/ja00730a036.

2. Mohamed M. Radwan, Suman Chandra, Shahbaz Gul, and Mahmoud A. ElSohly, "Cannabinoids, Phenolics, Terpenes and Alkaloids of Cannabis," *Molecules* 26, no. 2774 (May 8, 2021): 1, https://doi.org/10.3390/molecules 26092774.

3. Justin E. LaVigne, Ryan Hecksel, Attila Keresztes, and John M. Streicher, "Cannabis Sativa Terpenes Are Cannabimimetic and Selectively Enhance Cannabinoid Activity," *Scientific Reports* 11, no. 8232 (April 15, 2021): 11, https://doi.org/10.1038/s41598-021-87740-8.

4. Shimon Ben-Shabat, Ester Fride, Tzviel Sheskin, Tsippy Tamiri, Man-Hee Rhee, Zvi Vogel, Tiziana Bisogno, Luciano De Petrocellis, Vincenzo Di Marzo, and Raphael Mechoulam, "An Entourage Effect: Inactive Endogenous Fatty Acid Glycerol Esters Enhance 2-arachidonoyl-glycerol Cannabinoid Activity," *European Journal of Pharmacology* 353 (May 15, 1998): 30, https:// doi.org/10.1016/S0014-2999(98)00392-6.

5. Ethan B. Russo, "The Case for the Entourage Effect and Conventional Breeding of Clinical Cannabis: No 'Strain,' No Gain," *Frontiers in Plant Science* 9, article 1969 (January 2019): 1, https://doi.org/10.3389/fpls.2018.01969.

6. Anahad O'Connor, "Ask Well: Vitamin Expiration Dates," *The New York Times*, July 21, 2015, D6, https://well.blogs.nytimes.com/2015/07/20/ask-well -vitamin-expiration-dates/.

7. Pauline Lerner, "The Precise Determination of Tetrahydrocannabinol in Marihuana and Hashish," *United Nations Office on Drugs and Crime* (January 1, 1969): 41, https://www.unodc.org/unodc/en/data-and-analysis/bulletin/bul letin_1969-01-01_3_page007.html.

8. K. Narayanaswami, H. C. Golani, H. L. Bami, and R. D. Dua, "Stability of Cannabis Sativa L. Samples and Their Extracts, on Prolonged Storage in Delhi," *United Nations Office on Drugs and Crime* (January 1, 1978): 58, https://www.unodc.org/unodc/en/data-and-analysis/bulletin/bulletin_1978 -01-01_4_page007.html.

9. Magdalena Taschwer and Martin G. Schmid, "Determination of the Relative Percentage Distribution of THCA and Delta[9]-THC in Herbal Cannabis Seized in Austria: Impact of Different Storage Temperatures on Stability," *Forensic Science International* 254 (July 2015): 167, http://dx.doi.org/10.1016/j.forsciint.2015.07.019.

10. Taschwer and Schmid, "Determination of the Relative Percentage Distribution," 169.

11. Taschwer and Schmid, "Determination of the Relative Percentage Distribution," 170.

12. Luca Zamengoa, Chiara Bettina, Denis Badoccob, Valerio Di Marcob, Giorgia Mioloc, and Giampietro Frisona, "The Role of Time and Storage Conditions on the Composition of Hashish and Marijuana Samples: A Four-Year Study," *Forensic Science International* 298 (May 2019): 131, https://doi.org/10.1016/j.forsciint.2019.02.058.

13. Narayanaswami et al., "Stability of Cannabis sativa," 68.

14. Michael Starks, *Marijuana Chemistry: Genetics, Processing and Potency*, second ed. (Oakland, CA: Ronin Publishing, 1993), 14–15.

15. Zamengoa et al., "The Role of Time and Storage Conditions," 134.

16. Zamengoa et al., "The Role of Time and Storage Conditions," 133.

17. Zamengoa et al., "The Role of Time and Storage Conditions," 133.

18. Zamengoa et al., "The Role of Time and Storage Conditions," 136.

19. Robert Connell Clarke, *Marijuana Botany: An Advanced Study: The Propagation and Breeding of Distinctive Cannabis* (Berkeley, CA: And/Or Press, 1981), 153.

20. "Why Are Beer Bottles Brown?" O. Berk, accessed May 15, 2021, https://www.oberk.com/packaging-crash-course/why-are-beer-bottles-brown.

21. Zamengoa et al., "The Role of Time and Storage Conditions,"134.

22. K. P. Svoboda and T. Svoboda, "Herbs and Their Uses: Packaging and Storage," in *Encyclopedia of Food Sciences and Nutrition*, second ed., edited by Benjamin Caballero, Paul Finglas, and Fidel Toldra (Oxford, England: Academic Press, 2003), 3075, https://doi.org/10.1016/B0-12-227055-X/00591-5.

23. Clarke, *Marijuana Botany*, 154.

24. Jackie Bryant, "The Cannabis Industry's Plastic Problem," Healthline, October 30, 2020, https://www.healthline.com/health/cannabis-packaging#2-companies-are-getting-creative.

25. Avery N. Gilbert and Joseph A. DiVerdi, "Human Olfactory Detection of Packaged Cannabis," *Science and Justice* 60, no. 2 (March 2020): 170, https://doi.org/10.1016/j.scijus.2019.10.007.

26. Gilbert and DiVerdi, "Human Olfactory Detection," 170.

27. Gilbert and DiVerdi, "Human Olfactory Detection," 170.

28. Gilbert and DiVerdi, "Human Olfactory Detection," 171.

CHAPTER NINE

1. Juan Pablo Prestifilippo, Javier Fernández-Solari, Carolina de la Cal, María Iribarne, Angela M. Suburo, Valeria Rettori, Samuel M. McCann, and Juan Carlos Elverdin, "Inhibition of Salivary Secretion by Activation of Cannabinoid Receptors," *Experimental Biology and Medicine* 231, no. 8 (September 1, 2006): 1428, https://doi.org/10.1177/153537020623100816.

2. S. Joshi and M. Ashley, "Cannabis: A Joint Problem for Patients and the Dental Profession," *British Dental Journal* 220, no. 11 (June 10, 2016): 599, https://doi.org/10.1038/sj.bdj.2016.416.

3. Prestifilippo et al., "Inhibition of Salivary Secretion," 1421.

4. Joshi and Ashley, "Cannabis: A Joint Problem," 598.

5. Joshi and Ashley, "Cannabis: A Joint Problem," 600.

6. Fawad Javed, Abeer S. Al-Zawawi, Khaled S. Allemailem, Ahmad Almatroudi, Abid Mehmood, Darshan Devang Divakar, and Abdulaziz A. Al-Kheraif, "Periodontal Conditions and Whole Salivary IL-17A and -23 Levels among Young Adult Cannabis Sativa (Marijuana)-Smokers, Heavy Cigarette-Smokers and Non-Smokers," *International Journal of Environmental Research and Public Health* 17, no. 20, article 7435 (October 13, 2020), 7, https://doi.org/10.3390/ijerph17207435.

7. John Edward Swartzberg, Sheldon Margen, and the Editors of UC Berkeley Wellness Letter, *The Complete Home Wellness Handbook* (New York: Rebus Books, 2001): 287.

8. Mark Tambe Keboa, Ninoska Enriquez, Marc Martel, Belinda Nicolau, and Mary Ellen Macdonald, "Oral Health Implications of Cannabis Smoking: A Rapid Evidence Review," *Journal of the Canadian Dental Association* 86, (February 3, 2020): 6–7, https://jcda.ca/k2.

9. R. P. Antoniazzi, F. B. Lago, L. C. Jardim, M. R. Sagrillo, K. L. Ferrazzo, and C. A. Feldens, "Impact of Crack Cocaine Use on the Occurrence of Oral Lesions and Micronuclei," *International Journal of Oral and Maxillofacial Surgery* 47, no. 7 (July 2018): 894, https://doi.org/10.1016/j.ijom.2017.12.005.

10. Fernando Jose Guedes da Silva Júnior, Claudete Ferreira de Souza Monteiro, Thiago Alberto de Sousa Monteiro, Lorena Uchoa Portela Veloso, Larissa Alves de Araújo Lima, and Ludmila Kimbele Barbosa, "Oral Changes for Poly Drug Users: Multicenter Study," *International Archives of Medicine* 9, no. 146 (July 14, 2016): 6, https://doi.org/10.3823/2017.

11. Andrew Weil and Winifred Rosen, *From Chocolate to Morphine: Everything You Need to Know about Mind-Altering Drugs*, revised ed. (Boston: Houghton Mifflin, 2004), 137.

12. Peter Stafford, *Psychedelics Encyclopedia*, third ed. (Berkeley, CA: Ronin Publishing, 1992), 189.

13. Christine A. Northrop-Clewes and David I. Thurnham, "Monitoring Micronutrients in Cigarette Smokers," *Clinica Chimica Acta* 377, no. 1–2 (February 2, 2007): 14, https://doi.org/10.1016/j.cca.2006.08.028.

14. Northrop-Clewes and Thurnham, "Monitoring Micronutrients," 20.

15. Phyllis A. Balch, *Prescription for Nutritional Healing*, fourth ed. (New York: Avery, 2006), 709.

16. Balch, *Prescription for Nutritional Healing*, 17.

17. Balch, *Prescription for Nutritional Healing*, 708.

18. Northrop-Clewes and Thurnham, "Monitoring Micronutrients," 18.

19. Ross Trattler and Adrian Jones, *Better Healing through Natural Health*, second ed. (New York: McGraw-Hill, 2001), 433.

20. Balch, *Prescription for Nutritional Healing*, 24.

21. Northrop-Clewes and Thurnham, "Monitoring Micronutrients," 25.

22. Balch, *Prescription for Nutritional Healing*, 709.

23. Balch, *Prescription for Nutritional Healing*, 27.

24. Balch, *Prescription for Nutritional Healing*, 25.

25. Balch, *Prescription for Nutritional Healing*, 25.

26. Cynthia Aranow, "Vitamin D and the Immune System," *Journal of Investigative Medicine* 59, no. 6 (March 21, 2011): 881, http://dx.doi.org/10.2310/JIM.0b013e31821b8755, with full text at http://europepmc.org/backend/ptpmcrender.fcgi?accid=PMC3166406&blobtype=pdf.

27. Aranow, "Vitamin D," 882.

28. Northrop-Clewes and Thurnham, "Monitoring Micronutrients," 30.

29. Northrop-Clewes and Thurnham, "Monitoring Micronutrients," 29.

30. Balch, *Prescription for Nutritional Healing*, 38.

31. Northrop-Clewes and Thurnham, "Monitoring Micronutrients," 31.

32. Balch, *Prescription for Nutritional Healing*, 40.

33. Balch, *Prescription for Nutritional Healing*, 710.

34. T. Colin Campbell and Thomas M. Campbell, *The China Study*, second ed. (Dallas, TX: BenBella Books, 2005): 290–91.

35. Nicholas Wright, L. Wilson, M. Smith, B. Duncan, and P. McHugh, "The BROAD Study: A Randomized Controlled Trial Using a Whole Food Plant-Based Diet in the Community for Obesity, Ischemic Heart Disease or Diabetes," *Nutrition & Diabetes* 7, no. 3, e256 (March 2017): 8, https://doi.org/10.1038/nutd.2017.3.

36. Jo Robinson, *Eating on the Wild Side: The Missing Link to Optimum Health* (New York: Little, Brown, and Company, 2013), 5.

37. Robinson, *Eating on the Wild Side*, 5.

38. Kat Austin, "Juicing Cannabis: Medicine without the High," Key to Cannabis, July 28, 2019, https://keytocannabis.com/juicing-cannabis-medicine-without-the-high/.

39. "Resources," Cannabis International, accessed August 22, 2021, https://cannabisinternational.org/wordpress/index.php/resources/.

CHAPTER TEN

1. Donna Farhi, *The Breathing Book: Good Health and Vitality through Essential Breath Work* (New York: Henry Holt and Company, 1996), 83.

2. Kat Lay, "Air Pollution Blamed for 7M Deaths Every Year Worldwide," *The Times*, May 2, 2018, https://www.thetimes.co.uk/article/air-pollution -blamed-for-7m-deaths-every-year-worldwide-zd3fklt88.

3. CDC (U.S. Centers for Disease Control and Prevention), "CDC National Health Report Highlights," (2013): 8, https://www.cdc.gov/healthreport/publi cations/compendium.pdf.

4. Louis J. Aronne, "Obesity as a Disease: Etiology, Treatment, and Man-agement Considerations for the Obese Patient," *Obesity Research* 10, no. S12 (December 2002): 95S, https://doi.org/10.1038/oby.2002.201.

5. NIAAA (U.S. National Institute on Alcohol Abuse and Alcoholism), "Alcohol Facts and Statistics" (June 2021): 2, https://www.niaaa.nih.gov/pub lications/brochures-and-fact-sheets/alcohol-facts-and-statistics.

6. Robert S. Gable, "Comparison of Acute Lethal Toxicity of Commonly Abused Psychoactive Substances," *Addiction* 99, no. 6 (June 2004): 689, https://doi.org/10.1111/j.1360-0443.2004.00744.x, with full text at http://chem istry.mdma.ch/hiveboard/rhodium/pdf/psychoactives.acute.lethal.toxicity.pdf.

7. Andrew Weil and Winifred Rosen, *From Chocolate to Morphine: Everything You Need to Know about Mind-Altering Drugs*, revised ed. (Boston: Houghton Mifflin, 2004), 70.

8. Weil and Rosen, *From Chocolate to Morphine*, 78.

9. Cynthia Kuhn, Scott Swartzwelder, and Wilkie Wilson, *Buzzed: The Straight Facts about the Most Used and Abused Drugs from Alcohol to Ecstasy*, second ed. (New York: W.W. Norton, 2003), 135.

10. Christopher Cumo, "Cannabis" in *Encyclopedia of Cultivated Plants: From Acacia to Zinnia,* vol. 1, A–F, ed. Christopher Cumo (Santa Barbara, CA: ABC-CLIO, 2013), 204.

CHAPTER ELEVEN

1. National Academies of Sciences, Engineering, and Medicine, *Marijuana and Medicine: Assessing the Science Base* (Washington, DC: National Acad-emies Press, 1999), 126, https://doi.org/10.17226/6376.

2. Peter Gates, Adam Jaffe, and Jan Copeland, "Cannabis Smoking and Re-spiratory Health: Consideration of the Literature," *Respirology* 19, no. 5 (July 2014): 657, https://doi.org/10.1111/resp.12298.

3. Alison Mack and Janet Joy, *Marijuana as Medicine? The Science Beyond the Controversy* (Washington, DC: National Academies Press, 2001), 39, https://doi.org/10.17226/9586.

4. Jeanette M. Tetrault, Kristina Crothers, Brent A. Moore, Reena Mehra, John Concato, and David A. Fiellin, "Effects of Marijuana Smoking on Pulmonary Function and Respiratory Complications: A Systematic Review," *Archives of Internal Medicine* 167, no. 3 (February 12, 2007): 221, https://doi .org/10.1001/archinte.167.3.221.

5. Marcus H. S. Lee and Robert J. Hancox, "Effects of Smoking Cannabis on Lung Function," *Expert Review of Respiratory Medicine* 5, no. 4 (August 2011): 538, https://doi.org/10.1586/ers.11.40.

6. Donald P. Tashkin, "Effects of Marijuana on the Lung and Its Defenses against Infection and Cancer," *School Psychology International* 20, no. 1 (February 1999): 33, https://doi.org/10.1177/0143034399201003.

7. Lynn Zimmer and John P. Morgan, *Marijuana Myths, Marijuana Facts: A Review of the Scientific Evidence* (New York: Lindesmith Center, 1997), 116.

8. Tashkin, "Effects of Marijuana on the Lung," 25–26.

9. Tashkin, "Effects of Marijuana on the Lung," 24.

10. Kathryn Gracie and Robert J. Hancox, "Cannabis Use Disorder and the Lungs," *Addiction* 116, no. 1 (January 2021): 192, https://doi.org/10.1111/add .15075.

11. Donald P. Tashkin, "Smoked Marijuana as a Cause of Lung Injury," *Monaldi Archives for Chest Disease* 63, no. 2 (June 2005): 93, https://doi.org /10.4081/monaldi.2005.645, with full text at https://www.monaldi-archives .org/index.php/macd/article/view/645/633.

12. Donald P. Tashkin, "Marijuana and Lung Disease," *Chest Journal* 154, no. 3 (September 2018): 661, https://doi.org/10.1016/j.chest.2018.05.005.

13. Mehrnaz Ghasemiesfe, Brooke Barrow, Samuel Leonard, Salomeh Keyhani, and Deborah Korenstein, "Association between Marijuana Use and Risk of Cancer: A Systematic Review and Meta-Analysis," *Journal of the American Medical Association (JAMA) Network Open* 2, no. 11 (November 27, 2019): 11, https://doi.org/10.1001/jamanetworkopen.2019.16318.

14. Reena Mehra, Brent A. Moore, Kristina Crothers, Jeanette Tetrault, and David A. Fiellin, "The Association Between Marijuana Smoking and Lung Cancer: A Systematic Review," *Archives of Internal Medicine* 166, no. 13 (July 10, 2006): 1359, https://doi.org/10.1001/archinte.166.13.1359.

15. Gracie and Hancox, "Cannabis Use Disorder and the Lungs," 185.

16. Lee and Hancox, "Effects of Smoking Cannabis," 538.

17. Gates et al., "Cannabis Smoking," 655.

18. M. L. Lee, Milos Novotny, and K. D. Bartle, "Gas Chromatography/ Mass Spectrometric and Nuclear Magnetic Resonance Spectrometric Studies of Carcinogenic Polynuclear Aromatic Hydrocarbons in Tobacco and

Marijuana Smoke Condensates," *Analytical Chemistry* 48, no. 2 (February 1, 1976): 410–11, https://doi.org/10.1021/ac60366a048.

19. Robert Melamede, "Cannabis and Tobacco Smoke Are Not Equally Carcinogenic," *Harm Reduction Journal* 2, no. 1 (October 18, 2005): 2, https://doi.org/10.1186/1477-7517-2-21.

20. Melamede, "Cannabis and Tobacco Smoke," 3.

21. Michael R. Polen, Stephen Sidney, Irene S. Tekawa, Marianne Sadler, and Gary D. Friedman, "Health Care Use by Frequent Marijuana Smokers Who Do Not Smoke Tobacco," *Western Journal of Medicine* 158, no. 6 (June 1993): 596, https://www.ncbi.nlm.nih.gov/pmc/articles/PMC1311782/.

22. Polen et al., "Health Care Use by Frequent Marijuana Smokers," 597.

23. Zimmer and Morgan, *Marijuana Myths, Marijuana Facts*, 114.

24. Mary P. Martinasek, Jamie B. McGrogan, and Alisha Maysonet, "A Systematic Review of the Respiratory Effects of Inhalational Marijuana," *Respiratory Care* 61, no. 11 (November 1, 2016): 1549, https://doi.org/10.4187/respcare.04846.

CHAPTER TWELVE

1. Emilie Jouanjus, Valentin Raymond, Maryse Lapeyre-Mestre, and Valérie Wolff, "What Is the Current Knowledge about the Cardiovascular Risk for Users of Cannabis-Based Products? A Systematic Review," *Current Atherosclerosis Reports* 19, no. 26 (June 2017): 1, https://doi.org/10.1007/s11883-017-0663-0.

2. National Academies of Sciences, Engineering, and Medicine, *Marijuana and Medicine: Assessing the Science Base* (Washington, DC: National Academies Press, 1999), 121, https://doi.org/10.17226/6376.

3. William Holubek, "Medical Risks and Toxicology," in *The Pot Book: A Complete Guide to Cannabis*, ed. Julie Holland (Rochester, VT: Park Street Press, 2010), 146.

4. National Academies of Sciences, *Marijuana and Medicine,* 121.

5. Amitoj Singh, Sajeev Saluja, Akshat Kumar, Sahil Agrawal, Munveer Thind, Sudip Nanda, and Jamshid Shirani, "Cardiovascular Complications of Marijuana and Related Substances: A Review," *Cardiology and Therapy* 7, no. 1 (June 2018): 48, https://doi.org/10.1007/s40119-017-0102-x.

6. Robert L. Page, Larry A. Allen, Robert A. Kloner, Colin R. Carriker, Catherine Martel, Alanna A. Morris, Mariann R. Piano, Jamal S. Rana, and Jorge F. Saucedo, "Medical Marijuana, Recreational Cannabis, and Cardiovascular Health: A Scientific Statement from the American Heart Association,"

Circulation 142, no. 10 (September 8, 2020): e147, https://doi.org/10.1161 /CIR.0000000000000883.

7. Nicolas Rodondi, Mark James Pletcher, Kiang Liu, Stephen Benjamin Hulley, and Stephen Sidney, "Marijuana Use, Diet, Body Mass Index, and Cardiovascular Risk Factors (from the CARDIA Study)," *The American Journal of Cardiology* 98, no. 4 (August 2006): 482, https://doi.org/10.1016 /j.amjcard.2006.03.024.

8. Tarang Parekh, Sahithi Pemmasani, and Rupak Desai, "Marijuana Use among Young Adults (18–44 Years of Age) and Risk of Stroke: A Behavioral Risk Factor Surveillance System Survey Analysis," *Stroke* 51, no. 1 (January 2020): 310, https://doi.org/10.1161/STROKEAHA.119.027828.

9. Page et al., "Medical Marijuana, Recreational Cannabis, and Cardiovascular Health," e140.

10. Jouanjus et al., "What Is the Current Knowledge about the Cardiovascular Risk," 10.

11. Stephen Sidney, "Cardiovascular Consequences of Marijuana Use," *The Journal of Clinical Pharmacology* 42, no. S1 (November 2002): 64s, https:// doi.org/10.1002/j.1552-4604.2002.tb06005.x.

12. Ryan Vandrey, Annie Umbricht, and Eric C. Strain, "Increased Blood Pressure Following Abrupt Cessation of Daily Cannabis Use," *Journal of Addiction Medicine* 5, no. 1 (March 2011): 16, https://doi.org/10.1097 /ADM.0b013e3181d2b309, with full text at https://www.ncbi.nlm.nih.gov /pmc/articles/PMC3045206/.

13. Pál Pacher, Sándor Bátkai, and George Kunos, "Blood Pressure Regulation by Endocannabinoids and Their Receptors," *Neuropharmacology* 48, no. 8 (June 2005): 1130, https://doi.org/10.1016/j.neuropharm.2004.12.005.

14. Vandrey et al., "Increased Blood Pressure," 16.

15. Pacher et al., "Blood Pressure Regulation by Endocannabinoids," 1134.

16. National Academies of Sciences, *Marijuana and Medicine,* 121.

17. Holubek, "Medical Risks and Toxicology," 146.

18. Alexandre H. Watanabe, Leenhapong Navaravong, Thitipong Sirilak, Ratthanon Prasitwarachot, Surakit Nathisuwan, Robert L. Page, and Nathorn Chaiyakunapruk, "A Systematic Review and Meta-Analysis of Randomized Controlled Trials of Cardiovascular Toxicity of Medical Cannabinoids," *Journal of the American Pharmacists Association*, in press as of August 2021 (March 2021): S1544319121001114, https://doi.org/10.1016/j.japh.2021.03.013.

19. Dale Gieringer, email message to author, August 12, 2021.

20. Hassan Z. Khiabani, Jørg Mørland, and Jørgen G. Bramness, "Frequency and Irregularity of Heart Rate in Drivers Suspected of Driving under the Influence of Cannabis," *European Journal of Internal Medicine* 19, no. 8 (December 2008): 611, https://doi.org/10.1016/j.ejim.2007.06.031, with full text at https://www.sciencedirect.com/science/article/pii/S0953620508000654.

21. Khiabani et al., "Frequency and Irregularity of Heart Rate," 611.
22. Khiabani et al., "Frequency and Irregularity of Heart Rate," 608.
23. Vandrey et al., "Increased Blood Pressure," 17.

Works Cited

Abrams, Donald I., H. P. Vizoso, S. B. Shade, C. Jay, M. E. Kelly, and N. L. Benowitz. "Vaporization as a Smokeless Cannabis Delivery System: A Pilot Study." *Clinical Pharmacology & Therapeutics* 82, no. 5 (November 2007): 572–78. https://doi.org/10.1038/sj.clpt.6100200 with full text at: https://sci-hub.se/10.1038/sj.clpt.6100200.

Allen, J. H., G. M. de Moore, H. Heddle, and J. C. Twartz. "Cannabinoid Hyperemesis: Cyclical Hyperemesis in Association with Chronic Cannabis Abuse." *Gut* 53, no. 11 (November 2004): 1566–70. https://doi.org/10.1136/gut.2003.036350.

Antoniazzi, R. P., F. B. Lago, L. C. Jardim, M. R. Sagrillo, K. L. Ferrazzo, and C. A. Feldens. "Impact of Crack Cocaine Use on the Occurrence of Oral Lesions and Micronuclei." *International Journal of Oral and Maxillofacial Surgery* 47, no. 7 (July 2018): 888–95. https://doi.org/10.1016/j.ijom.2017.12.005.

Aranow, Cynthia. "Vitamin D and the Immune System." *Journal of Investigative Medicine* 59, no. 6 (March 21, 2011): 881–86. http://dx.doi.org/10.2310/JIM.0b013e31821b8755, with full text at http://europepmc.org/backend/ptpmcrender.fcgi?accid=PMC3166406&blobtype=pdf.

Aronne, Louis J. "Obesity as a Disease: Etiology, Treatment, and Management Considerations for the Obese Patient." *Obesity Research* 10, no. S12 (December 2002): 95S–96S. https://doi.org/10.1038/oby.2002.201.

Atapattu, Sanka N., and Kevin R. D. Johnson. "Pesticide Analysis in Cannabis Products." *Journal of Chromatography* 1612, article 460656 (February 8, 2020): 1–8. https://doi.org/10.1016/j.chroma.2019.460656.

ATSDR (Agency for Toxic Substances and Disease Registry, U.S. Centers for Disease Control and Prevention). "Public Health Statement for Propylene

Glycol." CAS#57-55-6 (September 1997): 1–3. https://www.atsdr.cdc.gov /toxprofiles/tp189-c1-b.pdf.

Austin, Kat. "Juicing Cannabis: Medicine without the High." Key to Cannabis, July 28, 2019. https://keytocannabis.com/juicing-cannabis-medicine-without -the-high/.

Azorlosa, J. L., M. K. Greenwald, and M. L. Stitzer. "Marijuana Smoking: Effects of Varying Puff Volume and Breathhold Duration." *The Journal of Pharmacology and Experimental Therapeutics* 272, no. 2 (February 1995): 560–69, https://www.ncbi.nlm.nih.gov/pubmed/7853169.

Backes, Michael. *Cannabis Pharmacy: A Practical Guide to Medical Marijuana.* New York: Black Dog & Leventhal Publishers, 2014.

Balch, Phyllis A. *Prescription for Nutritional Healing*, fourth ed. New York: Avery, 2006.

Bansal, Vasudha, and Ki-Hyun Kim. "Review of PAH Contamination in Food Products and Their Health Hazards." *Environment International* 84 (July 20, 2015): 26–38. https://doi.org/10.1016/j.envint.2015.06.016.

Ben-Shabat, Shimon, Ester Fride, Tzviel Sheskin, Tsippy Tamiri, Man-Hee Rhee, Zvi Vogel, Tiziana Bisogno, Luciano De Petrocellis, Vincenzo Di Marzo, and Raphael Mechoulam. "An Entourage Effect: Inactive Endogenous Fatty Acid Glycerol Esters Enhance 2-arachidonoyl-glycerol Cannabinoid Activity." *European Journal of Pharmacology* 353 (May 15, 1998): 23–31. https://doi.org/10.1016/S0014-2999(98)00392-6.

Bhatta, Dharma N., and Stanton A. Glantz. "Association of E-Cigarette Use with Respiratory Disease among Adults: A Longitudinal Analysis." *American Journal of Preventive Medicine* 58, no. 2 (February 2020): 182–90. https://doi.org/10.1016/j.amepre.2019.07.028.

Block, Robert I., Roxanna Farinpour, and Kathleen Braverman. "Acute Effects of Marijuana on Cognition: Relationships to Chronic Effects and Smoking Techniques." *Pharmacology Biochemistry and Behavior* 43, no. 3 (November 1992): 907–17. https://doi.org/10.1016/0091-3057(92)90424-E.

Bloor, Roger N., Tianshu S. Wang, Patrik Španěl, and David Smith. "Ammonia Release from Heated 'Street' Cannabis Leaf and Its Potential Toxic Effects on Cannabis Users." *Addiction* 103, no. 10 (October 2008): 1671–77. https:// doi.org/10.1111/j.1360-0443.2008.02281.x.

Braunstein, Mark Mathew. "A Connecticut Paraplegic Tells His Story: Marijuana Has Worked the Best in Easing Pain." *The Hartford Courant.* January 12, 1997, Sunday editorials section, C1, C4.

———. "First Aid for Cannabis Smokers: 10 Ways to Reduce the Health Risks of Smoking Marijuana." *Spirit of Change Magazine: Holistic New England* 29, no. 1 (Spring/Summer 2016): 22–27. https://www.SpiritofChange.org /Spring-2016/First-Aid-for-Cannabis-Smokers.

———. "Getting High and Staying Healthy: How to Reduce the Health Risks of Smoking Marijuana." *Treating Yourself: The Alternative Medicine Journal* 13 (Fall 2008): 55–64. http://treatingyourself.com/magazine/issue13.pdf.

Bryant, Jackie. "The Cannabis Industry's Plastic Problem." Healthline, October 30, 2020, https://www.healthline.com/health/cannabis-packaging#2 -companies-are-getting-creative.

Bureau of Cannabis Control (BCC) of the California Environmental Protection Agency, Department of Pesticide Regulation (DPR). https://cannabis.ca.gov /cannabis-regulations.

———. "Cannabis Batch Testing Certificate of Analysis." January 18, 2019. https://docs.google.com/viewer?url=https%3A%2F%2Fbcc.ca.gov%2Fclear %2Fdocuments%2Fweekly%2F20190122_update.xlsx.

———. "Cannabis Pesticides That Cannot Be Used." September 2018. https:// www.cdpr.ca.gov/docs/cannabis/cannot_use_pesticide.pdf.

———. "Medicinal and Adult-Use Cannabis Regulatory and Safety Act" (MAUCRSA). https://leginfo.legislature.ca.gov/faces/codes_displayexpand edbranch.xhtml?tocCode=BPC&division=10.&title=&part=&chapter=&arti cle=&nodetreepath=14.

Busse, Franziska P., Georg Martin Fiedler, Alexander Leichtle, Helmut Hentschel, and Michael Stumvoll. "Lead Poisoning Due to Adulterated Marijuana in Leipzig." *Deutsches Ärzteblatt International* 105, no. 44 (October 2008): 757–63. https://doi.org/10.3238/arztebl.2008.0757.

California Department of Food and Agriculture (CDFA), CalCannabis Cultivation Licensing, OCal Program. "Introducing the California Department of Food and Agriculture's OCal Program." https://www.cdfa.ca.gov/calcannabis /ocal.html.

Campbell, T. Colin, and Thomas M. Campbell. *The China Study*, second ed. Dallas, TX: BenBella Books, 2005.

Cannabis Certification Council's CCC Organically Grown Cannabis Certification. https://cannabiscertificationcouncil.org.

Cannabis International. "Resources." Accessed June 15, 2021. https://cannabis international.org/wordpress/index.php/resources/.

"Cannabis Research," Bedrocan International (website) accessed July 12, 2021, https://bedrocan.com/medicinal-cannabis/cannabis-research/.

Cannabis Safety and Quality Certification. https://www.csqcertification.com.

Cassidy, Francis. "PGR Weed Is Risky and Here's How to Spot It," RxLeaf, September 24, 2019. https://www.rxleaf.com/dangers-pgr-weed-identify -before-buy-medical-cannabis/.

CDC (U.S. Centers for Disease Control and Prevention). "CDC National Health Report Highlights." 2013. https://www.cdc.gov/healthreport/publica tions/compendium.pdf.

————. "Chemistry and Toxicology of Cigarette Smoke and Biomarkers of Exposure and Harm." Chapter 3 in *How Tobacco Smoke Causes Disease: The Biology and Behavioral Basis for Smoking-Attributable Disease*. Atlanta, GA: Centers for Disease Control and Prevention, 2010. https://www.ncbi.nlm.nih.gov/books/NBK53014/.

Certified Kind. https://www.certified-kind.com/certified-kind-rules.

Chadi, Nicholas, Claudia Minato, and Richard Stanwick. "Cannabis Vaping: Understanding the Health Risks of a Rapidly Emerging Trend." *Paediatrics & Child Health* 25, no. 1 (June 2020): S16–20. https://doi.org/10.1093/pch/pxaa016.

Clarke, Robert Connell. *Marijuana Botany: An Advanced Study: The Propagation and Breeding of Distinctive Cannabis*. Berkeley, CA: And/Or Press, 1981.

Clean Green Certified program. https://cleangreencertified.com.

Cozzi, Nicholas V. "Effects on Water Filtration on Marijuana Smoke: A Literature Review." *Newsletter of the Multidisciplinary Association for Psychedelic Studies (MAPS)* 4, no. 2 (1993). http://www.ukcia.org/research/EffectsOfWaterFiltrationOnMarijuanaSmoke.php.

Cumo, Christopher. "Cannabis" in *Encyclopedia of Cultivated Plants: From Acacia to Zinnia*, vol. 1, A–F, edited by Christopher Cumo. Santa Barbara, CA: ABC-CLIO, 2013.

Derudi, Marco, Simone Gelosa, Andrea Sliepcevich, Andrea Cattaneo, Domenico Cavallo, Renato Rota, and Giuseppe Nano. "Emission of Air Pollutants from Burning Candles with Different Composition in Indoor Environments." *Environmental Science and Pollution Research* 21, no. 6 (March 2014): 4320–30. https://doi.org/10.1007/s11356-013-2394-2.

————. "Emissions of Air Pollutants from Scented Candles Burning in a Test Chamber." *Atmospheric Environment* 55 (August 2012): 257–62. https://doi.org/10.1016/j.atmosenv.2012.03.027.

Doblin, Rick. "The MAPS / California NORML Water Pipe Study." *Newsletter of the Multidisciplinary Association of Psychedelic Studies (MAPS)* 5, no. 1 (Summer 1994). https://maps.org/news-letters/v05n1/05119wps.html.

Earlenbaugh, Emily. "Is Neem Oil Causing Cannabinoid Hyperemesis Syndrome?" Leafly, June 24, 2019. https://www.leafly.com/news/health/neem-oil-cannabinoid-hyperemesis-syndrome.

Earleywine, Mitch. "Pulmonary Harm and Vaporizers." In *The Pot Book: A Complete Guide to Cannabis*, edited by Julie Holland, 153–60. Rochester, VT: Park Street Press, 2010.

————. *Understanding Marijuana: A New Look at the Scientific Evidence*. Oxford, England: Oxford University Press, 2002.

Earleywine, Mitch, and Sara Smucker Barnwell. "Decreased Respiratory Symptoms in Cannabis Users Who Vaporize." *Harm Reduction Journal* 4, no. 11 (2007): 1–4. https://doi.org/10.1186/1477-7517-4-11.

Epperson, Anna E., Lisa Henriksen, and Judith J. Prochaska. "Natural American Spirit Brand Marketing Casts Health Halo around Smoking." *American Journal of Public Health* 107, no. 5 (May 2017): 668–70. https://doi.org /10.2105/AJPH.2017.303719, with full text at https://www.ncbi.nlm.nih .gov/pmc/articles/PMC5388969/.

Farhi, Donna. *The Breathing Book: Good Health and Vitality through Essential Breath Work.* New York: Henry Holt and Company, 1996.

FDA (U.S. Food and Drug Administration). "Applications for Premarket Review of New Tobacco Products." (September 2011): 1–23. https://www.fda .gov/files/tobacco%20products/published/PDF-Ver_Draft-Guidance-for-In dustry-Applications-for-Premarket-Review-of-New-Tobacco-Products.pdf.

———. "Harmful and Potentially Harmful Constituents in Tobacco Products; Established List; Proposed Additions." *Federal Register* 84, no. 150, Docket No. FDA-N-0143 (August 5, 2019): 38032–35. https://www.govinfo.gov /content/pkg/FR-2019-08-05/pdf/2019-16658.pdf.

Feldman, Jay, and Drew Toher. "Pesticide Use in Marijuana Production: Safety Issues and Sustainable Options." *Pesticides and You: A Quarterly Publication of Beyond Pesticides* 34, no. 4 (Winter 2014–15): 14–23. https://www .beyondpesticides.org/assets/media/documents/watchdog/documents/Pesti cideUseCannabisProduction.pdf.

Fine, Philip M., Glen R. Cass, and Bernd R. T. Simoneit. "Characterization of Fine Particle Emissions from Burning Church Candles." *Environmental Science & Technology* 33, no. 14 (July 1999): 2352–62. https://doi.org/10.1021 /es981039v.

Franciosi, Anthony. "Rolling Papers: The Ultimate Guide." Honest Marijuana Company. Accessed July 5, 2021. https://honestmarijuana.com/rolling-papers/.

Gable, Robert S. "Comparison of Acute Lethal Toxicity of Commonly Abused Psychoactive Substances." *Addiction* 99, no. 6 (June 2004): 686–96. https:// doi.org/10.1111/j.1360-0443.2004.00744.x, with full text at http://chemistry .mdma.ch/hiveboard/rhodium/pdf/psychoactives.acute.lethal.toxicity.pdf.

Gaoni, Yehiel, and Raphael Mechoulam. "Isolation and Structure of Delta-Tetrahydrocannabinol and Other Neutral Cannabinoids from Hashish." *Journal of American Chemistry* 93, no.1 (January 13, 1971): 217–24. https:// pubs.acs.org/doi/pdf/10.1021/ja00730a036.

Gargani, Yousef, Paul Bishop, and David W. Denning. "Too Many Mouldy Joints: Marijuana and Chronic Pulmonary Aspergillosis." *Mediterranean Journal of Hematology and Infectious Diseases* 3, no. 1 (January 13, 2011): 1–5. http://dx.doi.org/10.4084/MJHID.2011.005.

Gates, Peter, Adam Jaffe, and Jan Copeland. "Cannabis Smoking and Respiratory Health: Consideration of the Literature." *Respirology* 19, no. 5 (July 2014): 655–62. https://doi.org/10.1111/resp.12298.

Gauvin, David V., Zachary J. Zimmermann, Joshua Yoder, and Rachel Tapp. "Marijuana Toxicity: Heavy Metal Exposure through State-Sponsored Access to 'la Fee Verte.'" *Pharmaceutical Regulatory Affairs* 7, no. 1 (April 1, 2018): 1–10. https://doi.org/10.4172/2167-7689.1000202.

Geller, Andy. "Feds' Joint Effort May OK Weed as Rx for Ill." *New York Post*, March 18, 1999. https://nypost.com/1999/03/18/feds-j0int-effort-may-0k-weed-as-rx-f0r-ill.

Ghasemiesfe, Mehrnaz, Brooke Barrow, Samuel Leonard, Salomeh Keyhani, and Deborah Korenstein. "Association between Marijuana Use and Risk of Cancer: A Systematic Review and Meta-Analysis." *Journal of the American Medical Association (JAMA) Network Open* 2, no. 11 (November 27, 2019): 1–15. https://doi.org/10.1001/jamanetworkopen.2019.16318.

Gieringer, Dale. "Health Tips for Pot Smokers." In *Health Tips for Marijuana Smokers*, edited by Dale Gieringer, 20–23. San Francisco: California NORML, 1994.

———. "Marijuana Water Pipe and Vaporizer Study." *Newsletter of the Multidisciplinary Association for Psychedelic Studies (MAPS)* 6, no. 3 (Summer 1996): 59–66. https://maps.org/news-letters/v06n3/06359mj1.html.

Gieringer, Dale H. "Cannabis 'Vaporization': A Promising Strategy for Smoke Harm Reduction." *Journal of Cannabis Therapeutics* 1, no. 3-4 (2001): 153–70. https://www.cannabis-med.org/data/pdf/2001-03-04-9.pdf.

Gieringer, Dale, Joseph St. Laurent, and Scott Goodrich. "Cannabis Vaporizer Combines Efficient Delivery of THC with Effective Suppression of Pyrolytic Compounds." *Journal of Cannabis Therapeutics* 4, no. 1 (February 26, 2004): 7–27. https://doi.org/10.1300/J175v04n01_02, with full text at https://www.ukcia.org/research/CannabisVaporizer.pdf.

Gilbert, Avery N., and Joseph A. DiVerdi. "Human Olfactory Detection of Packaged Cannabis." *Science and Justice* 60, no. 2 (March 2020): 169–72. https://doi.org/10.1016/j.scijus.2019.10.007.

Goodman, Samantha, Elle Wadsworth, Cesar Leos-Toro, and David Hammond. "Prevalence and Forms of Cannabis Use in Legal vs. Illegal Recreational Cannabis Markets." *International Journal of Drug Policy* 76, article 10258 (February 2020): 1–10, https://doi.org/10.1016/j.drugpo.2019.102658.

Gracie, Kathryn, and Robert J. Hancox. "Cannabis Use Disorder and the Lungs." *Addiction* 116, no. 1 (January 2021): 182–90. https://doi.org/10.1111/add.15075.

Grover, Joel, and Matthew Glasser. "Pesticides and Pot: What's California Smoking?" NBC-TV Los Angeles, February 22, 2017. https://www.nbclo5angeles.com/news/i-team-marijuana-pot-pesticide-california/31341/.

Guedes da Silva Júnior, Fernando Jose, Claudete Ferreira de Souza Monteiro, Thiago Alberto de Sousa Monteiro, Lorena Uchoa Portela Veloso, Larissa Alves de Araújo Lima, and Ludmila Kimbele Barbosa. "Oral Changes for Poly Drug Users: Multicenter Study." *International Archives of Medicine* 9, no. 146 (July 14, 2016): 1–7. https://doi.org/10.3823/2017.

Harris, Bradford. "The Intractable Cigarette 'Filter Problem.'" *Tobacco Control* 20, no. 1 (April 18, 2011): i10–16. https://doi.org/10.1136%2Ftc.2010.040113.

Holmes, Mowgli, John M. Vyas, William Steinbach, and John McPartland. "Microbiological Safety Testing of Cannabis." *Cannabis Safety Institute* (May 2015): 16–17. https://cdn.technologynetworks.com/tn/Resources/pdf /microbiological-safety-testing-of-cannabis.pdf.

Holubek, William. "Medical Risks and Toxicology." In *The Pot Book: A Complete Guide to Cannabis*, edited by Julie Holland, 141–52. Rochester, VT: Park Street Press, 2010.

Ito, Hidemi, Keitaro Matsuo, Hideo Tanaka, Devin C. Koestler, Hernando Ombao, John Fulton, Akiko Shibata, Manabu Fujita, Hiromi Sugiyama, Midori Soda, Tomotaka Sobue, and Vincent Mor. "Nonfilter and Filter Cigarette Consumption and the Incidence of Lung Cancer by Histological Type in Japan and the United States: Analysis of 30-Year Data from Population-Based Cancer Registries." *International Journal of Cancer* 128, no. 8 (April 15, 2011): 1918–28. https://doi.org/10.1002/ijc.25531.

Javed, Fawad, Abeer S. Al-Zawawi, Khaled S. Allemailem, Ahmad Al-matroudi, Abid Mehmood, Darshan Devang Divakar, and Abdulaziz A. Al-Kheraif. "Periodontal Conditions and Whole Salivary IL-17A and -23 Levels among Young Adult Cannabis Sativa (Marijuana)-Smokers, Heavy Cigarette-Smokers and Non-Smokers." *International Journal of Environmental Research and Public Health* 17, no. 20, article 7435 (October 13, 2020), 1–10. https://doi.org/10.3390/ijerph17207435.

Jelsma, Martin, and Virginia Montañés. "Vicious Circle: The Chemical and Biological 'War on Drugs.'" *Transnational Institute's Drugs & Democracy Programme* (March 2001): 1–34. https://www.tni.org/files/download /viciouscircle-e.pdf.

Jett, James, Emily Stone, Graham Warren, and K. Michael Cummings. "Cannabis Use, Lung Cancer, and Related Issues." *Journal of Thoracic Oncology* 13, issue 4 (April 1, 2018): 480–87. https://doi.org/10.1016/j.jtho .2017.12.013.

Joshi, S., and M. Ashley. "Cannabis: A Joint Problem for Patients and the Dental Profession." *British Dental Journal* 220, no. 11 (June 10, 2016): 597–601. https://doi.org/10.1038/sj.bdj.2016.416.

Jouanjus, Emilie, Valentin Raymond, Maryse Lapeyre-Mestre, and Valérie Wolff. "What Is the Current Knowledge about the Cardiovascular Risk for Users of Cannabis-Based Products? A Systematic Review." *Current*

Atherosclerosis Reports 19, no. 26 (June 2017): 1–15. https://doi.org/10.1007/s11883-017-0663-0.

Keboa, Mark Tambe, Ninoska Enriquez, Marc Martel, Belinda Nicolau, and Mary Ellen Macdonald. "Oral Health Implications of Cannabis Smoking: A Rapid Evidence Review." *Journal of the Canadian Dental Association* 86, (February 3, 2020): 1–10. https://jcda.ca/k2.

Khan, Murad Ali, Abdul Wajid, Suhail Noor, Fareedullah Khan Khattak, Saeed Akhtar, and Inayat Ur Rahman. "Effect of Soil Contamination on Some Heavy Metals Content of Cannabis Sativa." *Journal of the Chemical Society of Pakistan* 30, no. 6 (December 2008): 805–9. https://jcsp.org.pk/issue Detail.aspx?aid=5d7c3bc9-8cfd-4194-a905-aa1f7a9c324e.

Khiabani, Hassan Z., Jørg Mørland, and Jørgen G. Bramness. "Frequency and Irregularity of Heart Rate in Drivers Suspected of Driving under the Influence of Cannabis." *European Journal of Internal Medicine* 19, no. 8 (December 2008): 608–12. https://doi.org/10.1016/j.ejim.2007.06.031, with full text at https://www.sciencedirect.com/science/article/pii/S0953620508000654.

Kollef, M. H. "Adult Respiratory Distress Syndrome after Smoke Inhalation from Burning Poison Ivy." *Journal of the American Medical Association (JAMA)* 274, no. 4 (July 26,1995): 358–59. https://doi.org/10.1001/jama.1995.03530040086059.

Kooy, Frank van der, B. Pomahacova, and R. Verpoorte. "Cannabis Smoke Condensate I: The Effect of Different Preparation Methods on Tetrahydrocannabinol Levels." *Inhalation Toxicology: International Forum for Respiratory Health* 20, no. 9 (October 2008): 801–4. http://doi.org/10.1080/08958370802013559.

Kornbluth, Jesse. "Poisonous Fallout from the War on Marijuana." *New York Times Magazine*, November 19, 1978. https://www.nytimes.com/1978/11/19/archives/poisonous-fallout-from-the-war-on-marijuana-paraquat.html.

Kuhn, Cynthia, Scott Swartzwelder, and Wilkie Wilson. *Buzzed: The Straight Facts about the Most Used and Abused Drugs from Alcohol to Ecstasy*, second ed. New York: W.W. Norton, 2003.

Lanaro, Rafael, José L. Costa, Silvia O. S. Cazenave, Luiz A. Zanolli-Filho, Marina F. M. Tavares, and Alice A. M. Chasin. "Determination of Herbicides Paraquat, Glyphosate, and Aminomethylphosphonic Acid [AMPA] in Marijuana Samples by Capillary Electrophoresis." *Journal of Forensic Sciences* 60, no. 1 (January 2015): S241–47. https://doi.org/10.1111/1556-4029.12628.

Landrigan, Philip J., Kenneth E. Powell, Levy M. James, and Philip R. Taylor. "Paraquat and Marijuana: Epidemiological Risk Assessment." *American Journal of Public Health* 73, no. 7 (July 1983): 784–88. https://ajph.apha publications.org/doi/pdf/10.2105/AJPH.73.7.784.

Lanz, Christian, Johan Mattsson, Umut Soydaner, and Rudolf Brenneisen. "Medicinal Cannabis: *In Vitro* Validation of Vaporizers for the Smoke-Free Inhalation of Cannabis." *Public Library of Science (PLOS)* 11, no. 1 (January 19, 2016): 1–18. https://doi.org/10.1371/journal.pone.0147286.

Larsson, Bonny K., Greger P. Sahlberg, Anders T. Eriksson, and Leif Á. Busk. "Polycyclic Aromatic Hydrocarbons in Grilled Food." *Journal of Agricultural and Food Chemistry* 31, no. 4 (1983): 867–73. https://pubs.acs.org/doi/pdf/10.1021/jf00118a049?casa_token=0WH6tvcFNWIAAAAA:r Jp6gOZEaaRliJ-Zt_lFp7ZNHXeKRbQqgV0MKCPuzvvapA9V6tskoX qqFVzcp8WITqL-aaDL6lBHdiZp.

Lau, Nicolas, Paloma Sales, Sheigla Averill, Fiona Murphy, Sye-Ok Sato, and Sheigla Murphy. "Responsible and Controlled Use: Older Cannabis Users and Harm Reduction." *International Journal of Drug Policy* 26, no. 8 (August 2015): 709–18. https://doi.org/10.1016/j.drugpo.2015.03.008, with full text at https://www.ncbi.nlm.nih.gov/pmc/articles/PMC4499492.

LaVigne, Justin, E. Ryan Hecksel, Attila Keresztes, and John M. Streicher. "Cannabis Sativa Terpenes Are Cannabimimetic and Selectively Enhance Cannabinoid Activity." *Scientific Reports* 11, no. 8232 (April 15, 2021): 1–15. https://doi.org/10.1038/s41598-021-87740-8.

Lay, Kat. "Air Pollution Blamed for 7M Deaths Every Year Worldwide." *The Times*, May 2, 2018. https://www.thetimes.co.uk/article/air-pollution -blamed-for-7m-deaths-every-year-worldwide-zd3fklt88.

Lee, M. L., Milos Novotny, and K. D. Bartle. "Gas Chromatography/Mass Spectrometric and Nuclear Magnetic Resonance Spectrometric Studies of Carcinogenic Polynuclear Aromatic Hydrocarbons in Tobacco and Marijuana Smoke Condensates." *Analytical Chemistry* 48, no. 2 (February 1, 1976): 405–16. https://doi.org/10.1021/ac60366a048.

Lee, Marcus H. S., and Robert J. Hancox. "Effects of Smoking Cannabis on Lung Function." *Expert Review of Respiratory Medicine* 5, no. 4 (August 2011): 537–47. https://doi.org/10.1586/ers.11.40.

Lerner, Pauline. "The Precise Determination of Tetrahydrocannabinol in Marihuana and Hashish." *United Nations Office on Drugs and Crime* (January 1, 1969): 39–42. https://www.unodc.org/unodc/en/data-and-analysis/bulletin /bulletin_1969-01-01_3_page007.html.

Lindblom, Eric. "Marijuana and Vaping: Shadowy Past, Dangerous Present." *The New York Times*, October 21, 2019. https://www.nytimes.com /2019/10/21/health/marijuana-and-vaping-shadowy-past-dangerous-present .html.

Loflin, Mallory, and Mitch Earleywine. "No Smoke, No Fire: What the Initial Literature Suggests Regarding Vapourized Cannabis and Respiratory Risk." *Canadian Journal of Respiratory Therapy* 51, no. 1 (Winter 2015): 7–9. https://www.ncbi.nlm.nih.gov/pmc/articles/PMC4456813/.

London, Jerome. "Paraquat Pot: The True Story of How the US Government Tried to Kill Weed Smokers with a Toxic Chemical in the 1980s." *Thought Catalog*, last modified February 4, 2021. https://thoughtcatalog.com/jeremy -london/2018/08/paraquat-pot.

Los Angeles City Attorney. "City Attorney Explains Medical Marijuana Issue on NBC." Los Angeles City Attorney Blogspot. October 13, 2009. http:// lacityorgatty.blogspot.com/2009/10/city-attorney-explains-medical.html.

Mack, Alison, and Janet Joy. *Marijuana as Medicine? The Science beyond the Controversy.* Washington, DC: National Academies Press, 2001. https://doi .org/10.17226/9586.

MacLean, Robert Ross, Gerald W. Valentine, Peter I. Jatlow, and Mehmet Sofuoglu. "Inhalation of Alcohol Vapor: Measurement and Implications." *Alcoholism: Clinical and Experimental Research* 41, no. 2 (February 2017): 238–50. https://doi.org/10.1111/acer.13291, with full text at https://www .ncbi.nlm.nih.gov/pmc/articles/PMC6143144/.

Mariani, John J., Daniel Brooks, Margaret Haney, and Frances R. Levin. "Quantification and Comparison of Marijuana Smoking Practices: Blunts, Joints, and Pipes." *Drug and Alcohol Dependence* 113, no. 2-3 (January 15, 2011): 249–51. https://doi.org/10.1016/j.drugalcdep.2010.08.008.

Martinasek, Mary P., Jamie B. McGrogan, and Alisha Maysonet. "A Systematic Review of the Respiratory Effects of Inhalational Marijuana." *Respiratory Care* 61, no. 11 (November 1, 2016): 1543–51. https://doi.org/10.4187 /respcare.04846.

McKeil, Jessica. "The Dangers of PGR Weed and How to Identify It," International HighLife, October 25, 2020. https://internationalhighlife.com/the -dangers-of-pgr-weed-and-how-to-identify-it.

McPartland, John M., and Ethan B. Russo. "Cannabis and Cannabis Extracts: Greater Than the Sum of Their Parts?" *Journal of Cannabis Therapeutics* 1, no. 3-4 (June 2001): 103–32. https://doi.org/10.1300/J175v01n03_08, with full text at www.cannabis-med.org/data/pdf/2001-03-04-7.pdf.

Medicinal Genomics Corporation. n.d. "Aspergillus: The Most Dangerous Cannabis Pathogen." Medicinal Genomics. Accessed August 20, 2021. https:// www.medicinalgenomics.com/aspergillus-dangerous-cannabis-pathogen/.

Mehra, Reena, Brent A. Moore, Kristina Crothers, Jeanette Tetrault, and David A. Fiellin. "The Association between Marijuana Smoking and Lung Cancer: A Systematic Review." Archives of Internal Medicine 166, no. 13 (July 10, 2006): 1359–67. https://doi.org/10.1001/archinte.166.13.1359.

Melamede, Robert. "Cannabis and Tobacco Smoke Are Not Equally Carcinogenic." *Harm Reduction Journal* 2, no. 1 (October 18, 2005): 1–4. https:// doi.org/10.1186/1477-7517-2-21.

Migoya, David, and Ricardo Baca. "Colorado Pot Industry Steps Up Pesticide Fight against Regulators." *The Denver Post*, May 1, 2016. https://www

.denverpost.com/2016/05/01/colorado-pot-industry-steps-up-pesticide-fight -against-regulators/

———. "Colorado Yields to Marijuana Industry Pressure on Pesticides," *The Denver Post*, October 3, 2015. https://www.denverpost.com/2015/10/03 /colorado-yields-to-marijuana-industry-pressure-on-pesticides/.

———. "Hickenlooper Issues Executive Order to Declare Tainted Pot a Threat to Public Safety," *The Denver Post*, October 2, 2016. https://www.denver post.com/2015/11/12/hickenlooper-issues-executive-order-to-declare -tainted-pot-a-threat-to-public/.

Mishra, Ajay, and Nikhil Dave. "Neem Oil Poisoning: Case Report of an Adult with Toxic Encephalopathy." *Indian Journal of Critical Care* 17, no. 5 (September-October 2013): 321–22. https://dx.doi.org/10.4103 %2F0972-5229.120330.

Montgomery, LaTrice, Erin A. McClure, Rachel L. Tomko, Susan C. Sonne, Theresa Winhusen, Garth E. Terry, Jason T. Grossman, and Kevin M. Gray. "Blunts versus Joints: Cannabis Use Characteristics and Consequences among Treatment-Seeking Adults." *Drug and Alcohol Dependence* 198 (May 2019): 105–111. https://doi.org/10.1016/j.drugalcdep.2019.01.041.

Montoya, Zackary, Matthieu Conroy, Brian D. Vanden Heuvel, Christopher S. Pauli, and Sang-Hyuck Park. "Cannabis Contaminants Limit Pharmaco-logical Use of Cannabidiol." *Frontiers in Pharmacology* 11, article 571832 (September 11, 2020): 1–10. https://doi.org/10.3389/fphar.2020.571832.

Munckhof, W. J., A. Konstantinos, M. Wamsley, M. Mortlock, and C. Gil-pin. "A Cluster of Tuberculosis Associated with Use of a Marijuana Water Pipe." *The International Journal of Tuberculosis and Lung Diseases* 7, no. 9 (September 1, 2003): 860–65. www.ingentaconnect.com/content/iuatld /ijtld/2003/00000007/00000009/art00009#.

Narayanaswami, K., H. C. Golani, H. L. Bami, and R. D. Dua. "Stability of Cannabis Sativa L. Samples and Their Extracts, on Prolonged Storage in Delhi." *United Nations Office on Drugs and Crime* (January 1, 1978): 57–69. https://www.unodc.org/unodc/en/data-and-analysis/bulletin/bulletin _1978-01-01_4_page007.html.

National Academies of Sciences, Engineering, and Medicine. "Butane." Chap-ter 1 in *Acute Exposure Guideline Levels for Selected Airborne Chemicals: Volume 12.* Washington, DC: National Academies Press, 2012. https://doi.org /10.17226/13377.

———. *The Health Effects of Cannabis and Cannabinoids: The Current State of Evidence and Recommendations for Research.* Washington, DC: National Academies Press, 2017. https://doi.org/10.17226/24625.

———. *Marijuana and Medicine: Assessing the Science Base.* Washington, DC: National Academies Press, 1999. https://doi.org/10.17226/6376.

NIAAA (U.S. National Institute on Alcohol Abuse and Alcoholism). "Alcohol Facts and Statistics." (June 2021):1–9. https://www.niaaa.nih.gov/publica tions/brochures-and-fact-sheets/alcohol-facts-and-statistics.

Nicholson, Kieran. "Denver Marijuana Cultivator Issues Statewide Recall over High Mold and Yeast Levels." *The Denver Post*, October 14, 2019. https:// www.denverpost.com/2019/10/14/denver-marijuana-recall.

Northrop-Clewes, Christine A., and David I. Thurnham. "Monitoring Micronu-trients in Cigarette Smokers." *Clinica Chimica Acta* 377, no. 1–2 (February 2, 2007): 14–38. https://doi.org/10.1016/j.cca.2006.08.028.

O. Berk. "Why Are Beer Bottles Brown?" accessed May 15, 2021. https:// www.oberk.com/packaging-crash-course/why-are-beer-bottles-brown.

O'Connor, Anahad. "Ask Well: Vitamin Expiration Dates." *The New York Times*, July 21, 2015. https://well.blogs.nytimes.com/2015/07/20/ask-well -vitamin-expiration-dates/.

Oeltmann, John E., Eyal Oren, Maryam B. Haddad, Linda K. Lake, Theresa A. Harrington, Kashef Ijaz, and Masahiro Narita. "Tuberculosis Out-break in Marijuana Users, Seattle, Washington, 2004." *Emerging Infec-tious Diseases* 12, no. 7 (July 2006): 1156–59. https://doi.org/10.3201 /eid1207.051436.

Okey, Sarah A. and Madeline H. Meier. "A Within-Person Comparison of the Subjective Effects of Higher vs. Lower-Potency Cannabis." *Drug and Alcohol Dependence* 216, article 108225 (November 2020): 1–8, https://doi .org/10.1016/j.drugalcdep.2020.108225.

Orecchio, Santino. "Polycyclic Aromatic Hydrocarbons (PAHs) in Indoor Emission from Decorative Candles." *Atmospheric Environment* 45, no. 10 (March 2011): 1888–95. https://doi.org/10.1016/j.atmosenv.2010.12.024.

Oregon Sungrown Farm Certification. https://www.oregonsungrown.org/osg -certification.

Pacher, Pál, Sándor Bátkai, and George Kunos. "Blood Pressure Regulation by Endocannabinoids and Their Receptors." *Neuropharmacology* 48, no. 8 (June 2005): 1130–34. https://doi.org/10.1016/j.neuropharm.2004.12.005.

Page, Robert L., Larry A. Allen, Robert A. Kloner, Colin R. Carriker, Catherine Martel, Alanna A. Morris, Mariann R. Piano, Jamal S. Rana, and Jorge F. Saucedo. "Medical Marijuana, Recreational Cannabis, and Cardiovascular Health: A Scientific Statement from the American Heart Association." *Cir-culation* 142, no. 10 (September 8, 2020): e131–52. https://doi.org/10.1161 /CIR.0000000000000883.

Pappas, R. Steve. "Toxic Elements in Tobacco and in Cigarette Smoke: In-flammation and Sensitization." *Metallomics* 3, no. 11 (November 2011): 1181–98. https://doi.org/10.1039/c1mt00066g.

Parekh, Tarang, Sahithi Pemmasani, and Rupak Desai. "Marijuana Use among Young Adults (18–44 Years of Age) and Risk of Stroke: A Behavioral Risk

Factor Surveillance System Survey Analysis." *Stroke* 51, no. 1 (January 2020): 308–10. https://doi.org/10.1161/STROKEAHA.119.027828.

Perez-Reyes, Mario. "Marijuana Smoking: Factors That Influence the Bioavailability of Tetrahydrocannabinol." *Research Findings on Smoking of Abused Substances*. NIDA Research Monograph 99 (1990): 42–62. http://citeseerx.ist.psu.edu/viewdoc/summary?doi=10.1.1.517.3186.

Peters, Jeremy, and Joseph Chien. "Contemporary Routes of Cannabis Consumption: A Primer for Clinicians." *The Journal of the American Osteopathic Association* 118, no. 2 (February 1, 2018): 67–70. https://doi.org/10.7556/jaoa.2018.020.

Polen, Michael R., Stephen Sidney, Irene S. Tekawa, Marianne Sadler, and Gary D. Friedman. "Health Care Use by Frequent Marijuana Smokers Who Do Not Smoke Tobacco." *Western Journal of Medicine* 158, no. 6 (June 1993): 596–601. https://www.ncbi.nlm.nih.gov/pmc/articles/PMC1311782/.

Prestemon, Jeffrey P., Frank H. Koch, Geoffrey H. Donovan, and Mary T. Lihou. "Cannabis Legalization by States Reduces Illegal Growing on US National Forests." *Ecological Economics* 164, article 106366 (October 2019). https://doi.org/10.1016/j.ecolecon.2019.106366.

Prestifilippo, Juan Pablo, Javier Fernández-Solari, Carolina de la Cal, María Iribarne, Angela M. Suburo, Valeria Rettori, Samuel M. McCann, and Juan Carlos Elverdin. "Inhibition of Salivary Secretion by Activation of Cannabinoid Receptors." *Experimental Biology and Medicine* 231, no. 8 (September 1, 2006): 1421–29. https://doi.org/10.1177/153537020623100816.

Pure Regenerative Cannabis Movement's Pure Certification. http://dempurefarms.com/pure-certification-agreement.

Radwan, Mohamed M., Suman Chandra, Shahbaz Gul, and Mahmoud A. ElSohly. "Cannabinoids, Phenolics, Terpenes and Alkaloids of Cannabis." *Molecules* 26, no. 2774 (May 8, 2021): 1–29. https://doi.org/10.3390/molecules26092774.

Ren, Meng, Zihua Tang, Xinhua Wu, Robert Spengler, Hongen Jiang, Yimin Yang, and Nicole Boivin. "The Origins of Cannabis Smoking: Chemical Residue Evidence from the First Millennium BCE in the Pamirs." *Science Advances* 5, no. 6 (June 12, 2019): eaaw1391. https://doi.org/10.1126/sciadv.aaw1391.

Rimington, J. "The Effect of Filters on the Incidence of Lung Cancer in Cigarette Smokers." *Environmental Research* 24, no. 1 (February 1981): 162–166. https://doi.org/10.1016/0013-9351(81)90142-0.

Robinson, Jo. *Eating on the Wild Side: The Missing Link to Optimum Health.* New York: Little, Brown, and Company, 2013.

Rodondi, Nicolas Mark James Pletcher, Kiang Liu, Stephen Benjamin Hulley, and Stephen Sidney. "Marijuana Use, Diet, Body Mass Index, and Cardiovascular Risk Factors (from the CARDIA Study)." *The American Journal of Cardiology* 98, no. 4 (August 2006): 478–84. https://doi.org/10.1016/j.amjcard.2006.03.024.

Root, Tik. "Cigarette Butts Are Toxic Plastic Pollution. Should They be Banned?" *National Geographic* (website). August 9, 2019. https://www.nationalgeographic.com/environment/article/cigarettes-story-of-plastic.

Rosenthal, Ed, with David Downs. *Marijuana Harvest: How to Maximize Quality and Yield in Your Cannabis Garden.* Piedmont, CA: Quick American Publishing, 2017.

Rosenthal, Ed, Dale Gieringer, and Tod Mikuriya. *Medical Marijuana Handbook: A Guide to Therapeutic Use.* Oakland, CA: Quick American Archives, 1997.

Rubenstein, Dana, Amanda Eisenberg, and Nick Niedzwiadek. "De Blasio's Marijuana Dreams Already Facing Headwinds in Albany." Politico, December 20, 2018. https://www.politico.com/states/new-york/albany/story/2018/12/20/de-blasios-marijuana-dreams-already-facing-headwinds-in-albany-761652.

Russo, Ethan B. "The Case for the Entourage Effect and Conventional Breeding of Clinical Cannabis: No 'Strain,' No Gain." *Frontiers in Plant Science* 9, article 1969 (January 2019): 1–8. https://doi.org/10.3389/fpls.2018.01969.

Russo, Ethan B., Chris Spooner, Len May, Ryan Leslie, and Venetia L. Whiteley. "Cannabinoid Hyperemesis Syndrome Survey and Genomic Investigation." *Cannabis and Cannabinoid Research* 10, no. 10 (July 5, 2021): 1–9. https://doi.org/10.1089/can.2021.0046.

Salthammer, Tunga, Jianwei Gu, Sebastian Wientzek, Rob Harrington, and Stefan Thomann. "Measurement and Evaluation of Gaseous and Particulate Emissions from Burning Scented and Unscented Candles." *Environment International* 155 (October 2021): 1–14. https://doi.org/10.1016/j.envint.2021.106590.

SC Labs (Science of Cannabis Laboratories). "Rolling Papers Tested for Heavy Metals and Pesticides." September, 2, 2020, 1–7. http://www.sclabs.com/wp-content/uploads/2020/09/SC-Labs-Report_Rolling_Papers_MKT00308.pdf.

Schauer, Gillian L., Brian A. King, Rebecca E. Bunnell, Gabbi Promoff, and Timothy A. McAfee. "Toking, Vaping, and Eating for Health or Fun: Marijuana Use Patterns in Adults, U.S., 2014." *American Journal of Preventive Medicine* 50, no. 1 (January 2016): 1–8, http://doi.org/10.1016/j.amepre.2015.05.027.

Schmidt, Elena. "PAH: This Is Why We Test Hemp and Cannabis for Polycyclic Aromatic Hydrocarbons." ACS Laboratory, August 5, 2020. https://acslabcannabis.com/blog/education/pah-this-is-why-we-test-hemp-cannabis-for-polycyclic-aromatic-hydrocarbons/#wild.

Seltenrich, Nate. "Cannabis Contaminants: Regulating Solvents, Microbes, and Metals in Legal Weed." *Environmental Health Perspectives* 127, no.8 (August 2019): 1–6. https://doi.org/10.1289/EHP5785.

———. "Into the Weeds: Regulating Pesticides in Cannabis." *Environmental Health Perspectives* 127, no. 4 (April 2019): 1–8. https://doi.org/10.1289/EHP5265.

Sidney, Stephen. "Cardiovascular Consequences of Marijuana Use." *The Journal of Clinical Pharmacology* 42, no. S1 (November 2002): 64s–70s. https://doi.org/10.1002/j.1552-4604.2002.tb06005.x.

Simonoetto, Douglas A., Amy S. Oxentenko, Margot L. Herman, and Jason H. Szostek. "Cannabinoid Hyperemesis: A Case Series of 98 Patients." *Mayo Clinic Proceedings* 87, no. 2 (February 2012): 114–19. https://doi.org/10.1016/j.mayocp.2011.10.005.

Singh, Amitoj, Sajeev Saluja, Akshat Kumar, Sahil Agrawal, Munveer Thind, Sudip Nanda, and Jamshid Shirani. "Cardiovascular Complications of Marijuana and Related Substances: A Review." *Cardiology and Therapy* 7, no. 1 (June 2018): 45–59. https://doi.org/10.1007/s40119-017-0102-x.

Spindle, Tory R., Edward J. Cone, Nicolas J. Schlienz, John M. Mitchell, George E. Bigelow, Ronald Flegel, Eugene Hayes, and Ryan Vandrey. "Acute Effects of Smoked and Vaporized Cannabis in Healthy Adults Who Infrequently Use Cannabis: A Crossover Trial." *Journal of the American Medical Association (JAMA)* 1, no. 7 (November 30, 2018): 1–14. https://doi.org/10.1001/jamanetworkopen.2018.4841.

Stafford, Peter. *Psychedelics Encyclopedia*, third ed. Berkeley, CA: Ronin Publishing, 1992.

Starks, Michael. *Marijuana Chemistry: Genetics, Processing and Potency*, second ed. Oakland, CA: Ronin Publishing, 1993.

Stone, Dave. "Cannabis, Pesticides and Conflicting Laws: The Dilemma for Legalized States and Implications for Public Health." *Regulatory Toxicology and Pharmacology* 69 (2014): 284–88. http://dx.doi.org/10.1016/j.yrtph.2014.05.015.

Sullivan, Nicolas, Sytze Elzinga, and Jeffrey C. Raber. "Determination of Pesticide Residues in Cannabis Smoke." *Journal of Toxicology* 2013, ID 378168 (May 2013):1–6. http://dx.doi.org/10.1155/2013/378168.

Sun+Earth Certified. https://www.certified-kind.com/sunearth-certified.

Svoboda, K. P., and T. Svoboda. "Herbs and Their Uses: Packaging and Storage." In *Encyclopedia of Food Sciences and Nutrition*, second ed., edited by Benjamin Caballero, Paul Finglas, and Fidel Toldra, 3071–77. Oxford, England: Academic Press, 2003. https://doi.org/10.1016/B0-12-227055-X/00591-5.

Swartzberg, John Edward, Sheldon Margen, and the Editors of UC Berkeley Wellness Letter. *The Complete Home Wellness Handbook* (New York: Rebus Books, 2001.

Taschwer, Magdalena, and Martin G. Schmid. "Determination of the Relative Percentage Distribution of THCA and Delta⁹-THC in Herbal Cannabis Seized in Austria: Impact of Different Storage Temperatures on Stability." *Forensic Science International* 254 (July 2015): 167–71. http://dx.doi .org/10.1016/j.forsciint.2015.07.019.

Tashkin, Donald P. "Effects of Marijuana on the Lung and Its Defenses against Infection and Cancer." *School Psychology International* 20, no. 1 (February 1999): 23–37. https://doi.org/10.1177/0143034399201003.

———. "Marijuana and Lung Disease." *Chest Journal* 154, no. 3 (September 2018): 653–63. https://doi.org/10.1016/j.chest.2018.05.005.

———. "Smoked Marijuana as a Cause of Lung Injury," *Monaldi Archives for Chest Disease* 63, no. 2 (June 2005): 93–100. https://doi.org/10.4081/mon aldi.2005.645, with full text at https://www.monaldi-archives.org/index.php /macd/article/view/645/633.

Taylor, Amelia, and Jason W. Birkett. "Pesticides in Cannabis: A Review of Analytical and Toxicological Considerations." *Drug Testing and Analysis* 12, no. 2 (February 2020): 180–90. https://doi.org/10.1002/dta.2747.

Tetrault, Jeanette M., Kristina Crothers, Brent A. Moore, Reena Mehra, John Concato, and David A. Fiellin. "Effects of Marijuana Smoking on Pulmonary Function and Respiratory Complications: A Systematic Review." *Archives of Internal Medicine* 167, no. 3 (February 12, 2007): 221–28. https:// doi.org/10.1001/archinte.167.3.221.

Trattler, Ross, and Adrian Jones. *Better Healing through Natural Health*, second ed. New York: McGraw-Hill, 2001.

V., Adrian. "Why Should You Avoid Bleached Rolling Papers?" May 7, 2017. Everyone Does It. Accessed July 5, 2021. https://www.everyonedoesit.com /blogs/blog/why-should-you-avoid-bleached-rolling-papers.

Valdes-Donoso, Pablo, Daniel A. Sumner, and Robin Goldstein. "Costs of Cannabis Testing Compliance: Assessing Mandatory Testing in the California Cannabis Market." *PLOS ONE* 15, no. 4 (April 23, 2020): 1–20. https:// doi.org/10.1371/journal.pone.0232041.

Van Dam, Nicholas T., and Mitch Earleywine. "Pulmonary Function in Cannabis Users. Support for a Clinical Trial of the Vaporizer." *International Journal of Drug Policy* 21, No.6 (November 2010): 511–13. https://doi .org/10.1016/j.drugpo.2010.04.001 with full text at: https://www.albany.edu /~me888931/Vaporizer.pdf.

Vandrey, Ryan, Annie Umbricht, and Eric C. Strain. "Increased Blood Pressure Following Abrupt Cessation of Daily Cannabis Use." *Journal of Addiction Medicine* 5, no. 1 (March 2011): 16–20. https://doi.org/10.1097

/ADM.0b013e3181d2b309, with full text at https://www.ncbi.nlm.nih.gov /pmc/articles/PMC3045206/.

Voltaire. *Candide.* New York: Boni & Liveright, 1918. https://gutenberg.org /ebooks/19942.

Wasson, Shirley J., Zhishi Guo, Jenia A. McBrian, and Laura O. Beach. "Lead in Candle Emissions." *Science of the Total Environment* 296, no. 1–3 (September 2002): 159–74. https://doi.org/10.1016/S0048-9697(02)00072-4.

Watanabe, Alexandre H., Leenhapong Navaravong, Thitipong Sirilak, Ratthanon Prasitwarachot, Surakit Nathisuwan, Robert L. Page, and Nathorn Chaiyakunapruk. "A Systematic Review and Meta-Analysis of Randomized Controlled Trials of Cardiovascular Toxicity of Medical Cannabinoids." *Journal of the American Pharmacists Association*, in press as of August 2021 (March 2021): S1544319121001114. https://doi.org/10.1016/j.japh.2021.03.013.

Waxman, Olivia B. 2017. "Bill Clinton Said He 'Didn't Inhale' 25 Years Ago." *Time Magazine*, March 29, 2017. https://time.com/4711887/bill-clinton-didnt -inhale-marijuana-anniversary/.

Weil, Andrew, and Winifred Rosen. *From Chocolate to Morphine: Everything You Need to Know about Mind-Altering Drugs*, revised ed. Boston: Houghton Mifflin, 2004.

Westervelt, Amy. "Chemical Enemy Number One: How Bad Are Phthalates Really?" *The Guardian*, February 10, 2015. http://www.theguardian.com /lifeandstyle/2015/feb/10/phthalates-plastics-chemicals-research-analysis.

Wilson, Tim. "The Wild West of Organic Cannabis." StratCann, February 10, 2021. https://stratcann.com/2021/02/10/the-wild-west-of-organic-cannabis/.

Wright, Nicholas, L. Wilson, M. Smith, B. Duncan, and P. McHugh. "The BROAD Study: A Randomized Controlled Trial Using a Whole Food Plant-Based Diet in the Community for Obesity, Ischemic Heart Disease or Diabetes." *Nutrition & Diabetes* 7, no. 3, e256 (March 2017): 1–10. https:// doi.org/10.1038/nutd.2017.3.

Zacny, James P., and L. D. Chait. "Breathhold Duration and Response to Marijuana Smoke." *Pharmacology Biochemistry and Behavior* 33, no. 2 (June 1989): 481–84. https://doi.org/10.1016/0091-3057(89)90534-0.

———. "Response to Marijuana as a Function of Potency and Breathhold Duration." *Psychopharmacology* 103, no. 2 (February 1991): 223–26. https://doi .org/10.1007/BF02244207.

Zamengoa, Luca, Chiara Bettina, Denis Badoccob, Valerio Di Marcob, Giorgia Mioloc, and Giampietro Frisona. "The Role of Time and Storage Conditions on the Composition of Hashish and Marijuana Samples: A Four-Year Study." *Forensic Science International* 298 (May 2019): 131–37. https://doi .org/10.1016/j.forsciint.2019.02.058.

Zarrabi, Ali J., Jennifer K. Frediani, and Joshua M. Levy. "The State of Cannabis Research Legislation in 2020." *New England Journal of Medicine* 382, no. 20 (May 2020): 1876–77. https://doi.org/10.1056/NEJMp2003095, with full text at https://www.ncbi.nlm.nih.gov/pmc/articles/PMC7302267/.

Zelinkova, Zuzana, and Thomas Wenzl. "The Occurrence of 16 EPA PAHs in Food: A Review." *Polycyclic Aromatic Compounds* 35, no. 2-4 (2015): 248–84. https://doi.org/10.1080/10406638.2014.918550.

Zimmer, Lynn, and John P. Morgan. *Marijuana Myths, Marijuana Facts: A Review of the Scientific Evidence.* New York: Lindesmith Center, 1997.

Index

abamectin, 88–89
Abrams, Donald I., 65–66
Air Quality Index (AQI), 100
alveoli cells, 4–5
animal experiments, 8–9, 52–53, 151–52
antioxidants, 130
anxiety, 149
apples, 44
arsenic, 98
aspergillus fungi, 94–95
azadirachtin, 90–91

BCC. *See* Bureau of Cannabis Control
beats per minute (BPM), 150
Bedrocan, 34
beeswax candles, 19
bifenazate, 88–89
black market, 60, 81–84, 89, 94, 98–99
blood pressure (BP), 147
blood pressure and heartbeat: animal experiment and smoking in, 151–52; BPM studies in, 150–51; cannabinoids and, 149; light and heavy smoking review studies on, 148; longtime and heavy tokers BP in, 149; position and posture abrupt change in, 149; smoking impact on, 147; stroke or heart attack danger and, 148–49; vital sign readings and "white-coat syndrome" in, 151
boiling points, 72–74
Booker, Cedella, 35
BP. *See* blood pressure
BPM. *See* beats per minute
Bradbury, Ray, 71
Braunstein, Mark, viii
breath, 3, 5–6, 135
Bureau of Cannabis Control (BCC), 87, 89, 94
butane-fueled lighters: cumulative toxic effects of, 15–16; short-and long-term effects of sniffing, 15
buyers guide: for herbal vaporizers, 70–71; for homegrown cannabis, 107

°C. *See* degrees Celsius
cadmium poisoning, 98

Canada, 31, 63, 86; CFIA organic
    certification in, 103; OG cannabis
    in, 103
Canada's Cannabis Act, 103
Canadian Food Inspection Agency
    (CFIA), 103, 104
cancer, viii, 142
candles: glass wand dangers in,
    20–21; health tip for pipes and,
    21; ingredients variety in, 19;
    smoldering and, 20; toothpicks
    and, 21; VOCs and PAH in, 19;
    waxes and fragrances study on,
    19–20; wicks health risks in, 20
cannabidiol (CBD), xvi, 69, 72–73,
    75; cannabis connoisseurs and,
    111; labels and percentage
    content in, 111–12; as primary
    cannabinoid, 110
cannabinoids, 34, 110, 149; boiling
    points of, 73; brain and salivary
    glands as receptors of, 127; filter
    tips loss of, 30–31; hand pipes
    tars and transfer of, 38–40; human
    lung linings and, 78; terpenes and,
    73; toking and loss of, 34; vaping
    and, 75; volatize temperatures of,
    72; water pipes and, 52
cannabis, 147; alternatives to
    smoking, xvi; ancient cultures
    use of, vii; black market, 82–83;
    Booker and personal joints
    of, 35; bud examination of,
    79; combustion temperatures
    of, 74; as communal or ritual
    experience, 35; conditions use
    of, vii; coughing and, 5, 7,
    143, 145; Earleywine on, 6;
    experiment number 2 and, 9;
    flame and volatize temperatures
    of, 72; health risk reduction in,
    xv, xvii; health tip for smokers

and, 5; on holding that toke, 4;
    ill effects minimization in, viii;
    inhalation and, vii–viii; inhale and
    exhale casually in, 3; journey and
    research of, viii–ix; lung cancer
    and COPD non-risk of, viii, 142;
    medical studies on breath and,
    5–6; medicinal benefits and safety
    profile of, vii; oregano analogy
    of, xvii; pathogens flourishing
    in, 5; physical ailments from,
    142; physical exercise and, 8;
    quick relief in, xvi; research on,
    31; respiratory illnesses and, 5;
    scientific studies on holding your
    breath and, 3; as slow burner, 27;
    "smoke-kiss" and second-hand
    smoke sharing in, 6; smoke risks
    and, xv–xvi; smoking as preferred
    method of, xvii; social acceptance
    growth of, xv; street lingo of, xvi;
    "tars" absorption and, 4; THC
    and CBD in, xvi; three ways of
    consuming, 127; tobacco mixing
    with, 26; traditional bud form
    survey of, xvi; underground code
    number for, 24; vaping flower
    recommendation of, viii
cannabis, home grown: buying guide
    for selecting, 107; first-party
    certification of, 105; industrialized
    or own hands carrot comparison
    in, 106; male reprobates in, 105;
    monks and nuns and shamans
    in, 106–7; success and failure in,
    105–6; warehouses versus home
    gardeners in, 106
cannabis, organically grown, 25;
    Canada and CFIA regarding,
    103; Cannabis Safety and
    Quality Certification program
    and, 105; CCC "Organically

Grown" Cannabis Certification program in, 104; Certified Kind and, 105; Clean Green Certified program and, 104; regulating and certifying of, 103; Sun+Earth Certified requirements for, 105; third-party certifiers and, 104

cannabis, potency preservation of: air defense storage tip for, 123; air exposure and experiment for, 118–19; airtight container choosing in, 119; airtight hard container for, 121; analysis listing on labels for, 112; camouflage and wasteful packaging of, 116–17, 120; cannabinoids identification in, 110; canning jars use in, 121; CBD and THC as primary cannabinoids in, 110; cold storage and, 116; condensation threat in, 116; Connecticut pharmacy vials and security in, 120; cool temperatures and, 112; culinary experts and oxidation in, 111; culinary herbs and spices and, 117; drug tolerance building in, 109; freezing and negative effects in, 115–16; heat reducing, 112; herbal grinder use in, 124; Italian study on, 113–14; labels and percentage content in, 111–12; light as destroyer of, 117; light control storage tip for, 118; light or air or heat debate in, 117–18; metal lids and, 121; mylar pouches for, 121, 122; nutritional supplements potencies listing and, 112; open container storage and, 118; oven bags for, 121; oxygen decomposition and, 118; PET and PP plastic use in,

119; plants and air and light and warmth in, 109; plastic drug vials and trichomes in, 119–20; prized batch preserving and results in, 115; pure flower seeking for, 109–10; refrozen and rethawed warning for, 116; silicone food storage bags for, 121, 122; storage tip for, 125; survivalists preparation for, 115; temperature control storage tip for, 117; THC depletion experiments and studies in, 112–13; traffic stops and odor sniffing research on, 122–23; trichomes damage control in, 116; UV ray exposure and, 117; year supply handling of, 124–25

cannabis, purity of: black-market quality and, 81; buying tip for, 89; cannabis law reform and, 102–3; chemical residue in smoke study and, 79–80; crop spraying and, 83–84; cultivation process chemicals and, 79; dealer whimsical yarns about, 80; female and male plants and, 80; fungicides and, 92–93; guerilla gardeners environment trashing and, 85; heavy metals and, 97–99; hit-and-run renegade farmers and, 85; home grown and, 105–7; home test kits and, 84; insecticides and, 87–89; local sources and, 82; microbes and, 93–97; neem oil and, 89–92; olfactory and visual inspection in, 81–82; online pot shop menus and, 83; organically grown and, 103–5; PAH and, 100–101; paraquat or glyphosate study in, 84–85; "paraquat pot" scare in, 83–84; pesticides and, 85–87;

PGRs and, 99–100; sandwich and freezer bags use in, 80; smoke aromas and, 82; terpenes richness in, 80; three natural components for, 82; unsavory substances in, 83; Washington Square Park adventure and, 81

Cannabis Certification Council (CCC), 104–5

cannabis hyperemesis syndrome (CHS), 90; azadirachtin poisoning in, 91; Russo research on, 91

cannabis law reform, 138; Big Cannabis regulation thwarting of, 102; community loss in, 103; grower property rights and, 102; home cultivation and Corporate Cannabis in, 102; "legalization and regulation" mantras of, 102

Cannabis Safety and Quality Certification program, 105

Cannabis sativa L., vii

canning jars, 121

CBD. *See* cannabidiol

CCC. *See* Cannabis Certification Council

cellulose acetate, 29–31

Certified Kind, 105

CFIA. *See* Canadian Food Inspection Agency

Cheap Vaporizer model, 63

chronic obstructive pulmonary disease (COPD), viii

CHS. *See* cannabis hyperemesis syndrome

"churchwarden pipe," 40

cigarette holders: pipe stems similarity to, 33; safety tip about, 34

cilia cells, 4–5

Clarke, Robert Connell, 96

Clean Green Certified program, 104

Clinton, Bill, 4

colds, 142–43

Connecticut, 119–20

Consumer Product Safety Commission, U.S. (CPSC), 119

COPD. *See* chronic obstructive pulmonary disease

coughing, 5, 7, 143, 145

CPSC. *See* Consumer Product Safety Commission, U.S.

crack smokers, 128

crop spraying, 83–84

DEA. *See* Drug Enforcement Agency, U.S.

degenerative diseases, 132–33

degrees Celsius (°C), 71–74

degrees Fahrenheit (°F), 71–74

the Doors (rock band), 4

The Doors of Perception (Huxley), 4

Drug Enforcement Agency, U.S. (DEA), 63

drug tolerance, 109

drug vials, tinted screw-top, 119

dry mouth: cannabinoid receptors in, 127; health tip to remedy, 129; salivary production decrease in, 128; THC and, 127

DuPont, 122

Earleywine, Mitch, 6, 9

e-cigarettes, 60

Edison, Thomas, 17

"entourage effect," 111, 133

Environmental Protection Agency (EPA), U.S., 55, 56, 88

European Union (EU), 101

eye irritation: alcoholic or caffeinated beverages avoidance for, 129; comfort tip to prevent, 129; home urine test and hydration for, 129

°F. *See* degrees Fahrenheit
Fahrenheit 451 (Bradbury), 71
fast food, 132
FDA. *See* Food and Drug
    Administration, U.S.
filter tips: cellulose acetate
    alternatives in, 31; corn husk
    or charcoal in, 31; health tip
    about, 31; Institute for Cancer
    Prevention study of, 30; lost
    cannabinoids in, 30–31; oxygen
    content increase in, 31; tobacco
    and, 29–30
flameless lighters: arc-shaped spark
    from, 17; descriptive names
    for, 16–17; health tip for using,
    18; technology of, 17; as Tesla
    lighters, 16; torch lighters as,
    17–18; USB charges and, 16
Food and Drug Administration, U.S.
    (FDA), 28, 55, 61, 104
fumes, 11, 15, 78
fungicides: fungus choice and,
    92; health tip for avoiding, 93;
    myclobutanil and hydrogen
    cyanide in, 92; myclobutanil
    indoor use as, 92–93; NBC-TV
    investigation regarding, 92; three
    month residue in, 93. *See also*
    microbes

Gieringer, Dale H., 64–65
glass, 20–21, 42–43, 47
goblet cells, 4–5
Goldberg, Rube, 64, 65
good health: air pollution and, 135;
    cannabis commending for, 138;
    cannabis smoking death rate
    and, 136–37; drug law reform
    and, 138; female and male
    breathing and, 135; gender-neutral
    respiration rate in, 135; medical

marijuana patient and side effects
    in, 137; near-perfect health and,
    136; pot legalization and criminal
    prosecution and, 137–38; society
    and cannabis reevaluation in,
    136; stress and peace of mind in,
    135–36; tobacco and obesity and
    alcohol deaths in, 136. *See also*
    blood pressure and heartbeat;
    lungs; vitamins and nutrients

hashish, 113
Health Canada, 86, 103, 104
heart attack, 148–49
heartbeat. *See* blood pressure and
    heartbeat
heat, 74, 76, 112, 117–18
heavy metals: absorption of, 97–98;
    contaminant limits to, 99; soil
    contamination of, 97
hemp, 20–21, 26–27, 31, 38, 103
herbal grinder, 124
"Hobbit pipes," 40
hotboxing and shotgunning, 53
Huxley, Aldous, 4
"hyperaccumulators," 98
hyperventilation, 7

ignition: butane-fueled lighters and,
    15–16; candle power in, 19–21;
    flameless lighters and, 16–18;
    hazmat surcharges and, 13; joint
    lighting and, 11–12; matchboxes
    and matchbook perils in, 13;
    odorless techniques mastering
    in, 12; piezo lighters and health
    tip for, 14–15; risky business of
    inhaling fumes from, 11; "safety
    matches" and "strike-anywhere
    matches" for, 12–13
insecticides, 87; abamectin
    and bifenazate as, 88–89;

contamination persistence of, 89;
EPA and bifenthrin as, 88; health
tip for heavy smokers and, 91–92;
insects and cannabis crops in, 88;
licensed and unlicensed growers
testing avoidance of, 89; Los
Angeles City Attorney's Office
spot check for, 88
Institute for Cancer Prevention, filter
tip study of, 30
Institute of Medicine (IOM), 24
Italian potency study (2019):
cannabis and hashish in, 113; four
different controlled environments
in, 114; results of, 114

joints, 76–77; avoid sharing of,
36; Booker and personal use of,
35; hand pipes similarity and
difference from, 46; health tip for
lighting, 18; lighting of, 11–12;
rolling paper and, 23
juiced raw cannabis, 134
junk food, 132

Kaiser Permanente Medical Center,
Oakland, California, 144

light, 109, 117–18
lighters, 14–15. *See also* butane-
fueled lighters; flameless lighters
Los Angeles City Attorney's Office,
88
lungs, viii, 61, 66, 78; alveoli cells
in, 4–5; cancer and cannabis in,
viii, 142; cannabis flower and
tobacco leaf comparison and, 143;
cannabis smoking and health of,
142; cannabis temporary damage
to, 146; cannabis use and medical
records reference and, 144–45;

capacity expansion and, 7–8;
clandestine potheads in study
and, 144; coughing and, 5, 7,
143, 145; DIY animal experiment
for, 8–9; dry nasal passages and,
145; goblet and cilia cells in, 4–5;
habitual smoking research and,
141–42; hyperventilation and, 7;
hypoxia and oxygen deprivation
in, 7; illness predicting and,
146; Kaiser medical records
technicians respiratory illness
study and results in, 144; Kaiser
report flaws and, 144, 145;
nonsmokers and colds in, 142–43;
smoke exposure and respiratory
diseases susceptibility in, 141;
smoke irritation in, 141; smokers
and colds in, 143; "systematic
studies" on, 145

Marley, Bob, 35, 80
matches, 12–13
Medicinal and Adult-Use Cannabis
Regulatory and Safety Act
(MAUCRSA), 87
mercury, 98
metric system, 71
microbes: aspergillus fungi and,
94–95; bacteria and handling
in, 94; cannabis grown without
fungicides health tip in, 96–97;
hydroponic growing and, 93–94;
mold and mildew spores and,
95–96; as pathogens, 93; viruses
and, 94; water and moisture in, 96
mold and mildew spores, 95–96
monks, 106–7
Moroccan *sepsi*, 43
myclobutanil, 92–93
mylar pouches, 121, 122

NBC-TV, 92

neem oil: azadirachtin toxin in, 90; CHS affliction and, 90–91; clinical studies and, 90; fields and greenhouses use of, 90; health tip for heavy smokers and, 91–92; insecticide add-ons and, 89; OMRI and, 90; organically based pesticides and, 90; poison ivy and, 90

nuns, 106–7

nutritional supplements, 112, 133

OCal Program, 104

OG. *See* organically grown

OMRI. *See* Organic Materials Review Institute

Oregon Sungrown Farm Certification, 104

organically grown (OG), 25, 103–5

Organic Materials Review Institute (OMRI), 90

oven bags, 121

oxygen, 7, 31, 118

PAH. *See* polycyclic aromatic hydrocarbons

paraffins, in candles, 19

"paraquat pot" scare, 83–84

passing out, 150

PEG. *See* polyethylene glycol

pesticides, 90; BCC guidelines and test results for, 87; California and, 86–87; code word for, 85; combustion process creation of, 87; Health Canada agency limits on, 86; other cides cover of, 86; state or federal laws limiting of, 86

PET. *See* polyethylene terephthalate

PG. *See* propylene glycol

PGRs. *See* plant growth regulators

piezo lighters, 14–15

pipes, hand, 18, 21, 34, 76–77; advantages of, 37; aluminum foil screen avoidance in, 44; apples and directions for use as, 44; ashes to ashes in, 46; baby bottle nipple use in, 42; Betty Boop's Grampy and thinking cap in, 37–38; bowl capping in, 38; bowl scrap out for, 46; brass or steel screens for, 44; cannabinoids and tars in, 39–40; cannabinoids transfer in, 38; "churchwarden pipe" or "Hobbit pipes" in, 40; cleaning drudgery of, 45–46; coin-shaped screens and, 44–45; corncob danger in, 43; cost savings of, 38; extra smoke and, 38; first-time long-stem smokers of, 39; flat-bottomed bowls use in, 43; glass hand pipes as crack pipes in, 43; gunk clean out for, 45; interchangeable mouthpiece for, 41–42; joints similarity and difference from, 46; as less hurried, 37, 38; as less irritating, 39; as less toxic, 38; as less wasteful, 38; long-stemmed benefits of, 40; long stem segment visual check for, 45; metal and glass stems of, 42; metal bowls in, 43; metal or wood stem use in, 40; own hybrid construction of, 43; pipe cleaners and, 40, 46; prehistoric ancestors and, 37; respiratory benefit of, 39; screen replacement in, 45; screen requirement for, 44; screens and coating burn off of, 45; segmented long-stemmed wooden pipe demonstration video in, 41; segments distribution for, 42;

sharing caution for, 41; soapstone and sandstone as, 43; stealth pipes and decoy drumsticks as, 41; stem cleaning for, 46; tars trapping of, 39; toothpick use for, 38; wooden bowls for, 42; wooden flute use as, 41

pipes, water, 18, 21, 34, 76–77; alcohol and, 51; alcohol wipes use for, 57; "animal" experiment for, 52–53; ash intake reduction for, 49–50; bacteria breeding environment in, 54; buy clear, 54; as cannabis culture accoutrements, 48; captured tar to captured cannabinoids ratio in, 52; chlorine bleach and, 50; cleaning procedures for, 55; cleanliness health and safety of, 54–55; coarse-grain salt and, 55; cold and hot water in, 50; dry storage for, 54; encrustation layer removal in, 56; harm reduction study on, 52; herbal vaporizers research shift in, 52; hot and dry smoke and, 48–49; hotboxing and shotgunning conduits in, 53; isopropyl alcohol use for, 55; mental well-being sense in, 48; 1993 and 1996 studies on, 51–52; non-chlorinated water use in, 50; particulate matter in, 49; research about, 51; respiratory diseases link to, 53–54; safe and legal alcohol disposal for, 56–57; as sculptural artform, 47; silicone or ceramic or glass models of, 47; smoke bubbles toxin trapping in, 49; smoke cooling of, 48; stoner lingo for, 47; TB risk factor in, 53–54; traditional tobacco use in, 47; urban air and ash in, 49;

vinegar or soap and hot water use in, 55; water change and, 50

plant growth regulators (PGRs): carcinogens in, 99; daminozide use as, 99–100; flower growth and, 99; paclobutrazol use as, 100; tips for avoiding, 100

poison ivy, 90

polycyclic aromatic hydrocarbons (PAH), 19; AQI registering of, 100; cannabis coating of, 101; as environmental toxin, 100; environment pervasiveness of, 101; EU limits on, 101; forest fire wood smoke forming of, 100; tips for avoiding, 101; wind dispersement of, 100–101

polyethylene glycol (PEG), 60

polyethylene terephthalate (PET), 119, 122

polypropylene (PP), 119, 123

posture, 149

propylene glycol (PG), 60–61

Pure Regenerative Cannabis Movement, 105

Reefer Madness, 13

respiratory illness, 5, 53–54, 141, 144

"roach," 29, 33–34

rolling paper: bleached, 25; colored and flavored papers avoidance in, 25; corner cutting of, 24; dependable burners for, 27; FDA requirements and, 28; filter tips and, 29–31; health tip for choosing, 28–29; hemp cultivation for, 26–27; IOM medicinal marijuana study and, 24; joints and, 23; last step and cotton swab use for, 35–36; lead and, 28; novices and, 24; OG claim on, 25; one sheet use of, 24; questionable ingredients in, 27–28; rice paper use as, 26; "roach" and, 29; roach clips and cigarette holders for, 33–34; SC Labs random testing of, 28; slow burners and free burners in, 27; smoking tips and, 32–33; sources variety of, 25; spliffs and blunts use as, 26; toking and, 34–35; traditional fibers for, 25; vegetable-based glues and, 25–26; YouTube videos about, 23–24

Rosenthal, Ed, 96

Russo, Ethan, 91

Safe Food for Canadians Act, 103

Science of Cannabis Laboratories (SC Labs), 28

selenium, 131

shamans, 106–7

shotgunning, 53

"smoke-kiss," 6

smoking tips: burn prevention in, 33; health and safety tips about, 33; make your own, 32; paper drinking straws as, 32–33

soy, in candles, 19

stroke or heart attack, 148–49

Sun+Earth Certified, 105

tallow, in candles, 19

tars, 4, 38–40, 52

TB. *See* tuberculosis

terpenes, 80; aroma absence in, 110–11; aromatic oils in, 110; boiling points of, 74; cannabinoids and, 73; "entourage effect" in, 111; Greek word root of, 110; human lung linings and, 78

Tesla, Nikola, 16

Tesla lighters, 16

tetrahydrocannabinol (THC), xvi, 51, 66, 69, 72–73, 75; cannabis connoisseurs and, 111; depletion experiments and studies on, 112–13; hashish and, 113; labels and percentage content in, 111–12; light and, 118; male plants and, 80; as primary cannabinoid, 110; salivation inhibiting of, 127

tobacco, 33–34, 136, 143, 147; additives and, 79; burn rate of, 11; cannabis mixing with, 26; cellulose acetate and, 29–30; e-cigarettes long-term study and, 60; Europe smoking practice of, 59–60; FDA regulating of, 104; filter tips and, 29–30; as free burner, 27; heavy metals in, 97; mentholated cigarettes and, 39; rolling papers and, 28; water pipes traditional use for, 47

toking, 4, 149; drag counting in, 35; Dutch study on, 34–35; hand and water pipes use in, 34; higher temperatures and, 35; side stream cannabinoids loss in, 34

tolerance, drug, 109

toothpicks, 20–21, 38, 46

torch lighters, 17–18

trichomes, 94, 97, 113, 115–16, 119–20, 122

tuberculosis (TB), 53–54

ultraviolet (UV) rays, 117

U.S. Department of Agriculture (USDA), 90, 105; food plants and toxic chemicals limiting of, 103; hemp seeds and, 103; OG status and, 103–4

U.S. Pharmacopeia, vii

UV. *See* ultraviolet rays

vaping oils: FDA classification of PG in, 61; health tip for using, 61; lung coating of, 61; PG and PEG use in, 60–61; solvent bathing in, 60

vaporizers, buyers guide for: cleaning ease of, 70; loading and unloading ease of, 70; long battery life and short recharging time of, 70; quick start-up times for, 70; temperature and variable temperature control in, 70–71

vaporizers, herbal, viii, 50, 52; abandonment of, 64; "boiling points" and, 72; buyers guide for, 70–71; Canada and, 63; cannabinoids delivery with, 75; cannabis waxes and oils and, 59; cannabis websites review caveat on, 69; competitive models in, 69; conduction mechanics of, 67–68; confusion surrounding, 59; convection mechanics of, 68; customers' enthusiasm shut-off of, 63; design flaws and, 77–78; e-cigarettes long-term study and, 60; efficiency variation of, 68; 8-session plan for, 74; first generation of, 63; Gieringer study on, 64–65; health selling point of, 76; health tips for, 77; heat goal of, 74; herb volatizing in, 62; history of, 63; human subject studies and, 76; hype of, 61–62; incremental temperature increase for, 74; joints and pipes versus, 76–77; less heat and irritation in, 76; lung health and, 66; medicinal use of, 75; metal oxides and other fumes in, 78; metric system and adjustable temperature controls of, 71; metric system

reader advisory for, 71; model choices for, 67; model sampling of, 68, 75–76; 1996 study of, 64; novelty tiring of, 78; online smoke shops video reviews about, 69; own health evaluation for, 77; remote adjustment of, 67; second generation models of, 64; significant innovations in, 66–67; smoking and vaping advantages in, 62; as "smolderizer," 62; solids to liquids boiling points and, 72–73; Swiss models study of, 66, 69; technology progress on, 65; test subjects and, 65; three-stage plan for, 75; 2004 research on, 65; 2007 pilot study of, 65–66; vaping oils and, 60–61; Volcano model of, 65, 98; word use in, 62

vegetable oil, in candles, 19

vitamins and nutrients: degenerative diseases and, 132–33; juiced raw cannabis and, 134; junk and fast food and, 132; nutritional supplements in, 133; phytonutrients and sources in, 134; smoking and loss of, 130; smoking depletion compensation in, 132; vitamin A and dietary sources in, 130; vitamin C and plant food in, 131; vitamin D and deficiency in, 131; vitamin E and organ protection in, 131

volatile organic compounds (VOCs), 19

Wall Street Journal, 21

War on (Some) Drugs, 63, 82, 84, 86, 145

Washington Square Park, Greenwich Village, 81

"white-coat syndrome," 151
whole foods diet, 133
wind dispersement, of PAH, 100–101

YouTube videos, 21, 23–24

zinc, 132

About the Author

Mark Mathew Braunstein is the author of five previous books on health, food, and drugs, including *Microgreen Garden* (2013) and *Sprout Garden* (1999). He has also contributed many dozens of articles to glossy magazines such as *Natural Health*, *Vegetarian Times*, and *Backpacker*. The author of *Good Girls on Bad Drugs*, he is a bad boy on a good drug. Since 1997, he has served as the poster child for medical marijuana in Connecticut, where he resides in Quaker Hill. As a paraplegic since 1990, his use of cannabis is medicinal for below the waist and is recreational for above. You can read his many articles and editorials about cannabis and medical marijuana at www.MarkBraunstein.org.